AF454146

Learning from Experience:
Memories of an Industrial Pharmacist

Learning from Experience: Memories of an Industrial Pharmacist

Prof. Manohar A. Potdar
President Technical,
Doshi Consultants Pvt. Ltd.,
Pharmaceutical Plant Design and Validation Consultants,
401, City-Centre, M.G. Road,
INDORE (M.P.) 452001.
Formerly,
Professor Emeritus,
Pharmaceutical Sciences,
Poona College of Pharmacy,
Bharati Vidyapeeth University,
Pune – 411038, India.

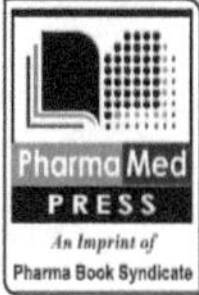

PharmaMed Press
An imprint of Pharma Book Syndicate

A Unit of BSP Books Pvt. Ltd.
4-4-309/316, Giriraj Lane,
Sultan Bazar, Hyderabad - 500 095.

Published by

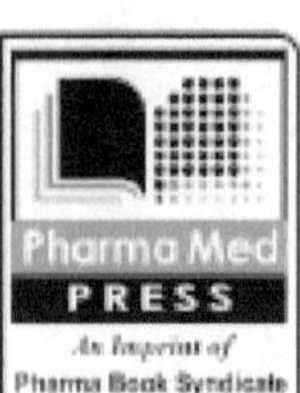

PharmaMed Press

An imprint of Pharma Book Syndicate

A Unit of BSP Books Pvt. Ltd.

4-4-309/316, Giriraj Lane, Sultan Bazar, Hyderabad - 500 095.
Phone: 040-23445605, 23445688; Fax: 91+40-23445611
E-mail: info@pharmamedpress.com

ISBN: 978-93-85433-72-6 (HB)

Foreword

I have been teaching M. Pharm students of Poona College of Pharmacy, Pune for the past seven years. I teach subjects like Quality Assurance, Plant Design, Validation, Quality Planning and Analysis, etc.

When I joined the college as a teacher in 2006, there were no syllabus oriented books for these subjects, so I started making notes both from the diverse books available to me and also using my own industrial experience as an industrial pharmacist for more than thirty-five years, obtained from both national and multinational organisations. Over a period of time I wrote three books based on these.

While teaching in the class I used to quote incidences from my industrial life as and when I found the situation to be appropriate. This helped the students visualize and imagine the exact situation when a particular theoretical aspect of the topic had to be applied. The narration of the incidences in the class used to take the students back into the same live environment, in which I had found myself sometime or the other in my industrial life. This not only used to make the subject interesting but made for the students sitting in the classroom environment, a very rich and useful experience for them.

This was going on for the last few years. Once in an internal meeting with my students along with the students of other colleges, studying the same subjects, some students of other colleges requested me to put my experiences on paper, so that these students who are not able to attend my classes will benefit from this. I seriously thought about this suggestion, liked the idea and finally made up my mind to put my pen on the paper for this purpose.

This book thus, is the result of this mental process of sharing some of my experiences from my personal industrial life, which include, both the serious side and the lighter vein too.

In most of the incidences I have written the names of the organisations, however at some places I have avoided it for obvious reasons. This however I have done without affecting the content of the message of the incidence.

I hope this scribbling will be of some use to the budding students of pharmacy and the upcoming industrial pharmacists. Happy reading friends.

Manohar A. Potdar

Acknowledgements

I am most grateful to many of my friends, my colleagues, my juniors and my seniors, who helped me develop myself into a successful industrial pharmacist and also evolve as an university teacher.

I am also grateful to my undergraduate and post graduate students with whom I spent my time sharing my industrial experiences. I always felt very comfortable with my students while sharing my success stories along with my failures and some blunders with an intention that they should learn from my experiences.

It is practically impossible to put on paper all those names, but still I would like to mention few of those names, who made a long lasting impression on my life. These are, Dr. S.G Patki, Dr. J.G Bhat, Ms Caroline Cabral, Dr. Ravi Rosha, Mr. V.P Samant, Mr Raghuvir Mangalurkar, Mr. A. Ramachandran, Mr. R Sridharan, Dr. Zach D' Souza, Mr. P.V Bhandarkar, Mr. S.M Desai, Mr. Bhaskar Patel, Dr. Prakash Khasgiwal and Mr. Anil Kumar Mishra. All these are my seniors in various companies. Some of my colleagues, I would like to mention are, Mr. Shyam Khante, Mr. P. Chatterjee, Mr. S.G Hardikar, OnkarNath Singh and Mr. Ajay Bhatia. And finally I would like to name some of my students whom I just cannot forget, for with these students I initially shared my experiences. They are, Ajit, Charu, Supriya, Shamita, Vibu, Parag, Ram, Jitendra, Shital, Sneha, Smridula, Nandu and Naresh.

Without my wife Manjari's encouragement, this book would not have seen the light of the day.

My student Smridula took all the efforts to convert my inlegible handwritten manuscript into a well formed book.

I am indebted to all of them.

Manohar A. Potdar

Contents

1

How I Landed into Pharmacy

Believe me, it was absolutely an accident. I was in second year B.Sc. class in Rajaram College, Kolhapur. Prakash Kulkarni alias Pakya was my classmate, friend and next door neighbour.

It was around 10 A.M. in the morning, I was getting ready to go to college. Usually Pakya and I used to leave our homes at about 10:30 A.M. every day. This meant that there was still about 30 min to go.

"Manya, Manya," Manya was my pet name in my friends circle. Pakya was calling me, standing on the road in front of my house.

"Pakya, what happened? It is just 10 o'clock."

"I know, but I have some interesting thing for you and of course also for me."

"What is it?"

"Come down and I will show you."

I went down through our wooden staircase, opened the main door and came out of my house.

"What is it yaar?"

"See this" Pakya had a local Marathi news-paper in his hand and was trying to show me something.

"What is that?" I asked again.

"You know at Karad, a town about 50 km from Kolhapur, where we stayed at that time, a new Pharmacy College is opening and an advertisement for admission has come."

"So?" I asked.

"So, we are going there right now by S.T. bus."

"And do what?"

"Try for admission yaar."

"And what about our B.Sc.?"

"Are you mad Manya? If we get admission to pharmacy, we will forget about the B.Sc. Yaar."

"What does this pharmacy actually mean?" my very innocent question to Pakya.

"I don't know, I really don't know."

"Then?"

"We first go to college and ask Rege sir, and then go to Karad. What do you say?"

"Are you crazy Pakya? You yourself don't know anything about what that pharmacy animal is like and you are telling me that we should take admission in that?"

"Yaar, listen, Manya. What are we going to do after B.Sc? Tell me?"

"And do you know exactly what we are going to do after pharmacy? Become a compounder or open a chemist's shop? Have you thought of anything? Pakya, you have really gone mad, let us continue with Rajaram College. Such a good college, you want to leave; do you really want to leave the company of Shoba, Sandhya, Rekha, Shraddha and all? No. No. I am not interested in all that."

I flatly refused.

"Yaar, Manya O.K. Come, let us go to college."

"Wait I'm coming." I said to Pakya, and went inside, took my notebook, apron and came out of my home.

"Aai, I am going to college." I shouted from the front door.

Throughout the way to college Pakya was trying to convince me, about the merits of pharmacy and demerits of B.Sc., even though he knew nothing about it.

We reached college, attended the first lecture of chemistry. Rege sir used to teach us chemistry. For a change we were sitting on the front bench that day. Pakya was uneasy. The bell rang. Rege sir closed his book, took the chalk and duster and started leaving the classroom.

Pakya suddenly got up from the bench, practically pulled me and ran behind Rege sir.

"Sir, Sir" Pakya called.

"Yes?" A big question mark was seen on Rege sir's face.

"Sir we want to talk to you for two minutes, can we?" Pakya requested.

"What do you want to talk about?"

"Just two minutes sir." Pakya answered.

"O.K. Come to my room."

"Thank you sir, thank you very much." Pakya profusely thanked Rege sir and we followed.

Rege sir entered his room, put his book, duster, chalk on his table. He just rubbed his palm to de-dust them and sat on the chair and said, "Yes, tell me."

"Sir, there is an advertisement in "Phudhari", the daily newspaper, about admission to Pharmacy college. We want to apply for it."

"So? Is this a good bye?"

"Sir, we really don't know about that course, we want to know you if it will be good to leave B.Sc. and go to pharmacy?" I tried to explain to Rege sir the reason we had come to his office.

He had put us both his hands on his face, and then slowly took them down, while slightly rubbing his face. He sat on the chair, relaxed a bit more, pushed the chair a little behind, probably stretched his legs under the table and said, "Oh. So that is the matter."

"Yes sir."

"See boys, Pharmacy Degree should be definitely better than B.Sc.. That's what I think. If you get admission, I think you should go for it." "Thank you, sir. Thank you very much. We will go and will let you know, what happens there," Pakya replied more than enthusiastically.

"Thank you sir," I replied.

"O.K." replied Rege sir, indirectly asking us to leave his room.

The only one single line advice of our beloved chemistry teacher in the college was a turning point in our lives.

Luck favoured us, we got admission and a totally new career in pharmacy started in August 1965.

2

THE FIRST JOB EVER

2nd June 1969, I landed in Mumbai in my uncle's house with my B. Pharm mark sheet and a provisional certificate stating that I have passed my B. Pharm examination with second class, from Shivaji University from Karad College of Engineering. Karad College of Engineering had a Pharmacy department at that time where we spent four years from Aug 1965 to April 1969.

My uncle was working in the Western Railway Head Office at Church Gate and we were staying in the Railway quarters in Vile Parke. We used to get 'Times of India' everyday in the house, and my uncle told me that every Wednesday and Saturday you get a lot of advertisements in the placement pages.

My uncle helped me to prepare a brief Bio-Data for me, and we started applying to every suitable advertisement that we used to read in the paper. It was simple, a standard letter was prepared as a model and we used to change only the details of the advertiser and the job described, sign that letter and attach a single page bio-data to that, put it in a white envelope, seal it and put a postal stamp on it and drop it in a post box.

Two to three weeks had passed, without any positive response. And then I started receiving some interview calls. Since I was applying for each and every type of job, I got calls for the position of medical representative, analysts, production chemists (That time the word pharmacist was not so popular even in the pharma industry and the pharmacists were also called as chemists.)

The days were passing; I was attending some interviews without achieving or trusting any real success.

I stayed in Kolhapur and studied in Karad, I really did possess the sophistication probably the Bombaites used to have at that time. We needed to compete with savvy students from U.D.C.T., L.M College of Pharmacy, Nagpur University. I was getting a little demoralised and depressed. But my uncle was a very good person; he used to motivate me and gave me some lessons, as to how to physically present yourself at the interview, how to converse in English effectively and so on.

Days were still passing and suddenly the day arrived, when I received a call letter a second time from the same company. When my uncle came in the evening, I told him that I received a call letter again. He was very happy. The second interview was after two days. I prepared myself to the best of my ability; I did not want to lose this opportunity.

I attended the interview with full confidence. And luck favoured me.

Dr. J.G. Bhatt, Head of the Q.C. Department in Merck-Sharp and Dohme finally told me that "Good, Manohar, we have selected you for the job of Q.C Technician for our Q.C lab. Please wait outside; you will receive the letter of appointment within half an hour O.K.?

"Yes sir, Thank you very much sir," I said as I profusely thanked him and left his office awaiting the letter.

After some time the receptionist called me and asked me to go to the personnel officer in the office. I went to his office; he was a very smart young man. "Sit down Mr. Potdar." He said.

"Thank you sir," I replied.

"Tell me, when you can report for duty?" he asked me.

I really did not know what to say but I replied, "Immediately sir."

He looked at me, smiled softly and said "This is your letter of appointment. Can you join on August 3rd?" and I replied "Yes sir, I will."

"Good." He said as he handed over the letter to me, smiled again and said, "See you on 3rd August at eight in the morning. O.K, Good luck."

I thanked him again and left the office and the factory. I was so excited; I had my first job ever in my hand.

3

ONE PAN BALANCE

It was 4th August 1969, just my second day in the new company. I had joined as Q.C. technician in the Q.C. Laboratory of Merck-Sharp and Dohme, in Mumbai.

It was not even 9 o'clock in the morning. I was in the lab with a new white apron and my boss Mr. Vengasarkar was showing me the lab. I was listening to him, and was a little apprehensive also. The lab was fairly large, with one small but separate instrument room, one microbiological media preparation area, one small glass ware washing area and so on.

Mr. Dave, who was our laboratory manager was sitting in one corner of the Lab, he had a separate table, a black landline phone along with an intercom. He was a tall, thin person, who mostly spoke in Gujrathi. Incidentally in our lab, we had around twenty analysts including two microbiologists, most of them were Gujrathi speaking. There were four "Senior Chemists" who were reporting to Mr. Dave our lab manager. Mr. Vengasarkar was one of those four, with whom I was supposed to be working in the raw material testing section.

"Manohar, come with me. We will go to the canteen, have our breakfast and then I will give you some analysis work in the lab." Mr. Vengasarkar told me.

"Yes sir," I replied as I followed him to the canteen as obediently.

We had our breakfast and came back to the lab. "Manohar, we have two samples of sodium chloride to be analysed." Vengasarkar gave me four small sample bottles containing sodium chloride of two batches. "The complete procedure is given in the I.P, you can follow that."

"Yes sir."

"Can you do that?" he tried to confirm.

"Yes sir"

"Anyway I'll show you some tests today, but then from tomorrow you have to do it yourself."

"Okay sir."

"Now you do one thing," Vengasarkar said to me, "take one of these bottles and weigh 500 mg on balance no. one over there." He showed me where balance number one was.

I kept one bottle on the table and took the other bottle in my hand and went to the balance.

There was a sturdy stool with a sand base in which a sophisticated weighing balance was kept. Another small revolving stool was there in front of the balance for the chemist. I went there, a little scared, my uneasiness and fear was clearly visible on my face, probably.

Mr. Vengasarkar was standing behind me, looking at what I was doing. But in fact I was doing nothing. I was standing still, and looking at the balance and also at the bottle in hand, alternatively.

"Manohar, sit on the revolving stool and weigh about 500 mg of the material from the bottle," Vengasarkar told me.

I sat down on the stool and started looking at the balance from all the sides. "What are you looking for?" Mr. Vengasarkar asked me in a slightly annoyed voice.

"Nothing sir, I am looking for the weighing pan sir." I said.

"Why? Can't you see the pan?" he asked. "Yes sir, I see that pan, I am looking for the second pan, I can't see that here." My voice and hand both were trembling as I said.

"What?" Vengasarkar literally shouted at me. I got scared. All the lab chemists also got a little scared, listening to Vengasarkar's loud voice.

Mr. Dave lifted his head slowly and looked at us and said, "What is the matter Vengasarkar?". "Nothing sir, nothing." Vengasarkar told him.

"Manohar, this is a one pan balance, have you not used this earlier?" he asked me. "I have never even heard of it sir." I answered innocently.

"Oh my god, you have never heard of one?

"No, Sir."

"Then what balances did you have in your lab, in the college?"

"Varanasi Sir."

"What Varanasi?"

"Varanasi two-pan balance Sir." I literally broke down. "I never used a one-pan balance sir." I admitted. "Oh! I don't know what to do with you. What type of B. Pharm degree do you have?" he said as he was totally annoyed. I was totally speechless; I really did not know what to say.

"Sir, why don't you leave it to me, I will explain it to him and show him how to use this balance. You don't worry Sir. I will show him." I heard a young girl chemist trying to calm Mr. Vengasarkar. I stood up from the stool and looked at her. I was literally in tears. I tried to control my tears and emotion, but failed. I held my lips tight and placed my left palm on my lips trying to control my sob.

"Okay, okay. Caroline, show him how to use it and make sure he doesn't spoil it," Mr. Vengasarkar told the girl who was trying to calm him.

Vengasarkar left the scene.

"Manohar, don't worry. Please sit down. I will show you how to use the one-pan balance." Caroline was very nice. I sat on the stool again.

She told me everything about the one-pan balance, how it works, how to use it, and what precautions should be taken. She also helped me by weighing one sample herself and asked me to weigh the other one. When I weighed the other one, I was very happy. I looked at her and said, "Thank you Caroline, thank you very much" with a vibrant but trembling voice.

She patted me on the shoulder and said, "Manohar don't worry, you will learn everything. I will teach you. If you need any help, don't go to anyone else. Ask me okay?"

"Okay," I replied as I wiped my eyes.

Caroline was a really good person. My entire stay at M.S.D was made not only comfortable, but enjoyable because of her. After more than forty years now, I still remember the incidence of the "One-pan balance" and my rescuer and most affectionate friend Caroline Cabral. She was actually a microbiologist. Presently she is settled in Singapore. You always meet some nice people in your life, whom you can never forget.

4

WATER ANALYSIS

In M.S.D. there was a style of giving analytical work to chemists. The freshers like me, were given analysis of sodium chloride, talcum, and similar inactive materials. Analysis of water used to be one of them.

One day I was analysing purified water for the first time. It had many tests and the last test on the list was loss on drying. I started carrying out tests one by one and when I came to the last test it was nearly four thirty in the evening. I weighed 100gms of water (nearly 100 ml) in a platinum crucible and kept it on a water bath for evaporation, it was four thirty by then. I was sitting on a stool there, waiting for this 100 ml of water to evaporate.

Everyone was preparing to leave, because the lab used to close by five. Caroline looked towards me and saw that I was still sitting on the stool. She asked me, "Hey man, are you not planning to go home today?"

"I have yet to complete this last test, loss on drying test." I replied.

"What? LOD you are doing it now? It will take up to seven to complete the analysis, are you going to wait here until then?"

"I don't know, but what else can I do?"

She laughed.

"Why are you laughing?" I asked Caroline.

"You fool, this test should be done right at the beginning, at nine in the morning, that's why I am laughing."

"Why?" I asked innocently, "It is the last test in the specification." I continued.

"So what? It is not necessary that you need to do the tests in the same order as they are given there. If you do this test first then you can do the other tests simultaneously. You should put the water for evaporation and simultaneously perform the other tests, so that by eleven or so you can weigh the dried crucible and note the gain in weight. You need not do it at a quarter to five. You understand?"

I realised my mistake and asked, "So what can I do now?"

"Do you have the sample of water?"

"Yes I do."

"Close it tightly and keep it inside with a proper label." she stopped the water batch as she was saying this. She threw the water from the crucible in the sink and deposited the platinum crucible to the lab locker.

"Now listen, tomorrow first thing when you come in the morning put the LOD sample. Okay?"

"Yes"

"Now go run, change your apron otherwise you will miss your bus."

"Thank you Carol." I ran to catch the bus.

Next day she showed me how to rearrange the sequence of tests for a product and start analysis. She gave me a simple guide line for starting any analysis. It was something like this:

1. Collect the samples for tomorrow's analysis from the senior chemist at about four in the evening.

2. Make a small check list of the materials required for analysis e.g.,

   - Normal solutions
   - Molar solutions
   - Indicators
   - Glassware required
   - Any specific glassware or accessories needed like iodine flask, platinum crucible etc.

3. First thing in the morning check the sequence of the tests, collect everything required near you, particularly the specific glassware. See that all the reagents required for the tests are in stock, if not then inform the person who makes the reagent solution and standardises it in advance so that no time is wasted.

Apart from these she also gave a few other small suggestions. This really improved my work.

I thanked Caroline for all her advice and she replied with a warm smile.

5

LEAVING THE FIRST JOB

Things were going smoothly at work. The Q.C job by now had become okay for me. I learned the basic skills required as a Q.C technician. My colleagues in the lab were good. My equation with my boss, Mr. Vengasarkar developed into a good bond. I found, in fact that he was a really good boss. Even though, initially I thought otherwise.

My friend Caroline; remained helpful to me throughout my term at the company. I just cannot forget her.

Most of my industry friends, those who passed out from our Karad college were working in the Pharma-Production, some were in F.D.A and a few left for U.S.A. Whenever we met each other in one of Mumbai's many hotels, we used to talk about our jobs. Though I had a job, I was not really enjoying it. All of my friends who were in production were thoroughly enjoying their jobs. I always had a liking for production but since I got my first job in Q.C and also the salary was good; four hundred rupees a month, which was considered to be a good salary during the late sixties. The monthly expenses did not exceed two hundred rupees and so I used to send two hundred rupees home every month.

One day my classmate Anil Gupte met me at our CIBA stop and said, "Manohar, are you interested in production?"

"Why not?" I exclaimed.

"We have two vacancies in CIBA."

"That is good yaar Anil; tell me what should I do?"

"Nothing, make an application on a plain paper addressed to "The Production Manager-CIBA" and give it to me tomorrow evening without fail."

"Okay. You will get it tomorrow evening positively. What are you going to do with that?"

"Don't worry I will give it to Dr S.J. Pataki, in fact he was asking 2-3 days ago, if I know any good candidate." "Good yaar, please do it for me. I will definitely give you the paper tomorrow. Okay." "Okay," he answered.

The bus started. I waved my hands. Things went very smoothly and I got my second job order in my hand as, "Assistant Pharmacist-Production."

I got a resignation letter typed from my uncle, who was very good at English drafting, and gave it to Dr J.G. Bhat, our Quality Control Head. He accepted it without any hesitation. My lab colleagues arranged a small send off in a hotel at Vile-Parle. My colleagues had also purchased a small gift. After the send-off was over, Rajendra Khanderia handed over the gift pack to Dr. Bhat for presenting it to me. He took it, looked at it and also looked at the gathering and handed over the gift pack to Caroline.

"Caroline, please come here and give the gift to your friend Manohar." Dr. Bhat said to Caroline. Everyone was a little surprised and that surprise was palpable on everyone's face.

"Come, come Caroline, I want you to present the gift to your friend. Am I right Caroline?"

"Thank you, sir." Caroline replied as she took the gift pack from Dr. Bhat.

Caroline handed over the gift pack to me and at that moment we looked into each other's eyes. I was unable to utter a single word. Rajendra clicked a photograph.

Caroline asked me to open the gift pack, I did. It was a nice, small, small handy, Agfa click III camera which I preserved carefully till I retired from my service in the year 2005, a long span of 36 years. I, unfortunately, lost it in the flood of 26th July, 2005 in Badalpur.

I was very happy to join CIBA, as a Production Chemist, because I wanted to be in production. But was I happy to leave M.S.D? My Q.C lab? My Caroline? Probably not. But life is, unpredictable. To meet is an accident but to part is nature.

I left M.S.D to join CIBA in the production department, but what I had learned in M.S.D's Q.C lab, I had not learnt in six years of my college life, two years in science college and four years in pharmacy college. Some of the things I learnt were;

1. How to use a pipette? Why the bulb should be held by the thumb and why to close the sucking end by a finger.

2. Why the spectrophotometer, cuvette should be held in the fingers from the opaque side.

3. Importance of time.

4. How and why to be helpful? However what I did not understand at that time was why Caroline had helped me.

5. And the most important and funny thing was how to use a one-pan balance.

6

JOB OF A PRODUCTION MAN

Somewhere in February, March of 1970 I joined CIBA in its cosmetics manufacturing department, where my colleague Anil Gupte was working. Anil was my classmate for four years of Pharmacy.

When I joined CIBA I did not know which department I would be joining. I only knew that I would be in production. I was in fact very keen to work in some areas like tablets, capsules or injections, but when I was put in cosmetics i.e., Binaca section, I was not very happy. The only good thing was Anil Gupte was with me in the same section. This section had three areas namely, toothpastes, creams and powders.

A few days after joining, I once met Dr. S.J. Patki, who had done his PhD from UK and was our Production Head, a very decent and sober boss. I requested him to transfer me from cosmetics to pharmaceutical production.

I was in his office standing in front of him.

"Yes Manohar, tell me why do you want to change from cosmetics to pharmaceuticals? Tell me," he asked. "Sit down, sit down," he added.

"Sir, I am a pharmacist and want to work in pharmaceutical manufacturing rather than cosmetics," I replied.

"What will happen because of this?" He asked.

"I like that Sir," I continued.

"Manohar, please remember, that as a production man, the job in every department is the same. You need to plan the work, you have to supervise the workers working in the section, you have to keep production records, you have to see that your department is well maintained, see that you meet the production plan of the month and so on. Now tell me what you are doing in the Binaca section? Whatever you are doing in the Binaca section, your other friends are doing in the other departments. Only difference is that they are manufacturing tablets, liquids and injections while you are manufacturing cosmetics. Don't you realise that in fact you have an unusual opportunity to learn something which your friends don't. Production is after all production. Everyone has a great scope to come up in life, if they have the talent and I know for certain that you have it."

I was listening very carefully to what Dr Patki was saying, and I realised that even if I was working in the Binaca section I will achieve everything that I am capable of. Those fifteen-twenty minutes in the room of Dr. Patki, changed my thinking about looking at cosmetics and pharmaceuticals differently. I was of the opinion that manufacture of cosmetics was somewhat inferior to manufacturing of pharmaceuticals. But after that talk I was convinced that it was not. Today I realise how great and humane Dr. Patki was. He never scolded or shouted at me. He allowed me to speak my mind about my grievance and in the most sober manner he convinced me.

I left his room with satisfaction. "Thank you sir, thank you very much. I will remember your advice," I said while leaving his room.

"Manohar, if you still feel you should work in pharma section, I will transfer you at the next available opportunity," he said.

But I never went back to him. I started enjoying my job, my colleagues and my role.

7

WRONG ADDITION

I worked in CIBA till July 1971 i.e. about 16 months only, during this period, I made one major mistake in manufacturing. I saw one great mistake committed by my colleague in the liquid department. I also saw some heart touching incidences.

The cosmetics department and ointment department were very close to each other. The Binaca section Head was Mr. Naik and ointment section Head was Mr. Shaha. Sometimes if Mr. Shaha was absent I used to go there and make a batch of ointment. Mr. Shaha had taught me the three or four ointments that we were involved in manufacturing there.

It was a regular day as any other. I came to my section, Mr. Naik told me, "Manohar, Mr. Shaha is not coming today, you ask Anil to look after your production and you go to the ointment section. Anand is there, you take the scheduled batch of ointment. Okay?"

"Yes sir," I said and I went to the ointment section. Anand was there, he was the worker in the ointment section.

"Anand we have to take the batch."

"Yes sir, the material for two batches is there in the department. Sir, Mr Shaha told me yesterday, which product is to be taken, I will start heating the pan sir, for melting the base," Anand told me.

"Okay," I said.

In the day store, that day there was material for two products. So there was material for two different products, two different batches.

We started manufacturing the product. The two pallets of two different products were kept side by side. (Actually these should have been sufficiently segregated. But unfortunately, they were not.)

We made the base, filtered it while hot and kept it on slow stirring for cooling.

"Anand I am going to the wash room. I will return soon. See that the chilled water and stirrer is on."

I came back after about 15-20 minutes. I saw that Anad was mixing the drug in the base. Being a regular worker he used to proceed with the work even in the absence of a supervisor. (Not at all a good manufacturing practice.)

"What are you doing Anand?" I asked.

"Mixing the drug sir," he replied.

We used to get the drug in double polythene bags with the label in between the two bags. We were supposed to keep the labels of each of the batches together and finally attach these labels to the B.P.C.R. Each label was required to be signed by the supervising pharmacist.

"Where is the label?" I asked.

"I have kept it in the drawer sir," he said

I opened the drawer and took out the label for signing and I was shocked by what I saw. The label was not of the drug that we were supposed to be manufacturing a product of. Anand had definitely made a mistake picking the drug from the other palette and added it and mixed it into the base also. The bases for both the products were different. There was no practical way to recover the batch. I was extremely afraid of the situation.

"Anand, stop that and come here," I literally shouted at him.

"What happened sir?" Anand was got scared hearing my voice.

"Anand you have added the wrong drug to the base. Do you know that?"

"Oh my god. What do we do now?"

"I don't know. I don't know," I said very seriously. "The drug or the batch, both cannot be recovered Anand."

"It has never happened in the past especially by me sir. I really don't know how this mistake happened." Anand was literally in tears.

"Anand let us go to Mr. Naik and tell him about what has happened, we have to tell him. We have no choice Anand." I was equally scared. We went to Mr. Naik and told him the whole episode and he was also helpless.

"Stop the batch at once," Mr. Naik said. We went back to the department, stopped the chilling and mixing and were waiting in the department, literally shaken and waiting to know what was going to happen.

By now Dr. Patki and Mr. Naik entered the department. We were standing in one corner.

"Yes, what happened Manohar?" Dr. Patki asked me.

I briefly explained the situation.

"You know you have to be very careful in manufacturing Manohar?"

"Yes sir."

"Anand, you are an experienced operator, how could you make such a mistake?"

"Sorry sir, I really don't know how I made this mistake," Aanad replied.

"Mr. Naik, call Dr Dalal from R and D and see if anything could be done to salvage this batch, and let me know. Anand, remove the batch from the pan and kept it aside. Collect the raw materials for both the batches and keep them separately under quarantine. Let us see what can be done," said Dr. Patki and left the scene.

Two days later we realised that nothing could be done with that batch and the batch was destroyed in the presence of Dr. Vora, our Q.C Head at that time.

On the third day at about 4 o' clock Dr. Patki called Mr. Naik, Anand and I into his office.

Anand and I received a formal letter of warning. "Manohar and Anand, both of you have to be more careful in your work in the future. This time the management has not taken a serious action against you but see that this does not happen again. You must understand that ultimately it is a major loss for the company. Please be more careful in the future," he repeated.

"Sorry sir, it will never happen again." Both of us replied in a mild and trembling voice. We left the cabin of Dr. Patki and went down.

This was the first mistake in my career as a manufacturing pharmacist. It gave me a very sound lesson, NEVER NEGLECT YOUR DUTY. It was Dr. Patki, who was a highly matured and humane person and that is why he explained the seriousness of the mistake without demoralising us. I understood the first principle of management, give an opportunity to a person to correct himself, do not demotivate him and he will improve.

8

DROPPING THE GLASS THERMOMETER IN THE PAN

When I was working in CIBA, I was attached to the Binaca section and occasionally I used to work in the ointment section.

It was a regular day just like any other, I was in the ointment department where Anand had melted and filtered the base and had kept it in an open pan for cooling. There was a small stirrer stirring the cooling base.

The active substance was supposed to be added when the temperature of the base comes to less than 50 °C. we had a glass thermometer with which we used to check the temperature, by dipping the glass thermometer into the cooling ointment base. (Murder of cGMP) I wanted to know what the temperature of the base was, so I dipped the thermometer into the base and started looking at the base. Anand was doing something behind me and accidently bumped into me from behind, the thermometer slipped form my hand and slipped down slowly into the congealing molten base. I did not know what to do. I looked back and said, " Anand yaar, what are you doing?"

"What happened sir?"

"You bumped into me and the thermometer slipped from my hand and that bloody thing is gone down and sitting at the bottom of the pan." I replied in an annoyed voice.

Anand immediately stopped the stirrer. We started looking into the pan to locate the thermometer. The base was hazy and we could not see the thermometer. Anand got a long stainless steel rod and slowly started to feel for the thermometer inside the pan. The ointment base was getting thicker because it was cooling down.

Finally after a lot of efforts we were able to take out the thermometer from the ointment base.

"Thank god." Anand said.

"Wait Anand, we have to see whether the thermometer is intact or not, then only we can thank god."

Anand washed the thermometer. We were quite lucky. The bulb as well as the stem of the thermometer was absolutely intact. The situation was saved.

The lesson that was learnt from this incident, was never dip a thermometer in the main vessel to check the temperature. You may take out a sample to check the temperature. Of course nowadays none of these situations arise as there are highly advanced temperature sensing devices available.

9

"OTRIVIN" FAILURE

Otrivin was an external liquid preparation. Mr. Vijay Shinde, the liquid formulation pharmacist used to manufacture that preparation. He was a very senior pharmacist in CIBA at that time. One day he started to manufacture a batch, the batch was filtered, and he was to start with the next step i.e., filling of the batch. He then received a phone call from his home asking him to return home immediately as his wife had suddenly taken ill. He had no choice but to leave.

He came to our Binaca section and told Mr. Naik, our Binaca section Head that "Please ask someone to look after the 'Otrivin' batch. I have already sent a sample to the Q.C lab. Sunila is analysing it. The result will be available by 10 o'clock or so. Once the result is received, continue filling the bottles, of which twenty thousand have already been washed and kept ready. Hegade, the filling operator knows all about this. Please do this for me as I have to rush home, since my wife is not well."

"Okay, okay. Don't worry Vijay. I will look into that," Mr. Naik said and Vijay rushed home.

"Manohar, please go to the Q.C lab and check with Sunila if the otrivin batch has been released for filling or not. And if it has been released then ask Hegade to start filling. Okay?"

"Yes sir," I replied and made my way to the Q.C lab.

"Sunila, is the Otrivin liquid batch released? We want to start the filling process," I said to her.

"Yes, yes. You can start the filling process. It has been released. I will send the report half an hour later," Sunila said.

I came down to the liquid department, and asked Hegade to start the filling process. The bottles were ready for filling; the solution was okay for assay and pH, so there was no issue. Hegade was a senior operator and charge hand. He quickly arranged the filling line and started the filling and sealing operation. I once again confirmed that twenty thousand bottles were ready for filling and ROPP caps for sealing.

"Hegade, I am going to the Binaca section. If you want anything call me. I am there. See that the filling volume is properly adjusted to 10 ml and check in between too." I instructed him before I left and went to my department.

The filling operation was going on well. I checked the volume 3 or 4 times during filling. At about 4:30 P.M. Hegade came to me and said, "Sir, we have run out of bottles, but some solution is still remaining. I need more bottles to fill."

"What? The bottles are over but the solution is still there? What are you saying? We had 20,000 bottles. Normally we require only 19,800 bottles. How can it be that the bottles are over? Please check once again and tell me," I told Hegade.

"No sir, I have checked everything, we have run out of bottles." he confidently told me.

"The volume filled was alright no? Has the volume filled ever been less than 10 ml?"

"No sir, I have seen to that and you have also checked in between. The volume was never less than 10 ml. I am sure sir." He was really confident.

"Come then let us go and see what has gone wrong." Hegade and I went to the Otrivin filling line.

Everything was okay. The fact remained that still about 5-6 litres of solution still remained in the container. How did this happen? The assay was also correct, then what had gone wrong?

Mean while Mr Naik had come on scene and we explained the situation to him.

"Who analysed the bulk Manohar?"

"Sunila, Sir."

"Okay. Just come with me."

Mr. Naik and I went up to the Q.C lab. "Sunila, the otrivin batch assay was alright when you analysed it in the morning?" Mr. Naik asked.

"Why Sir? Any problem?"

"Yes, we are facing some problem. Can you show me your workbook?"

Mean while Mr. Deshpande, our assistant Q.C manager had come over to us.

"What is the matter Mr. Naik?" he asked.

"Deshpande Saab, we have filled 20,000 bottles of Otrivin, with the correct fill volume, and yet we are left over with some solution. According to me the only probability is the volume of the bulk solution is more by about 5 to 6 litres somehow. But if the assay is correct, then something must be wrong somewhere, we are unable to get to the point." Mr. Naik explained.

Sunila brought her workbook.

"Was there any issue in the assay, Sunila?" Mr. Deshpande asked.

By now Sunila was in a bad shape. "Sir actually the assay was slightly less, but it never happened in the past. I only analyse the Otrivin all the time," Sunila said to Mr. Deshpande.

"If the assay was less then why did you release the batch?"

"Sir actually I thought it must be my mistake in the analysis and Manohar wanted to start filling so I released the batch."

"And what does your written report say?"

"I have not yet made it Sir."

"Tell me, what was your original reading?"

By now Mr. Deshpande was a little annoyed with her. He took the workbook and quickly calculated the assay and found that it was low.

"Mr. Naik, please hold the batch and immediately place under quarantine, the batch stands rejected. On the face of it, it looks like the volume adjustment and assay both were wrong."

"Okay Sir." Mr. Naik and I came down and quarantined the batch.

The whole batch was recovered and reprocessed, afterwards.

The lesson we inferred from this incident;

- Never take anything for granted.
- Have confidence in your work, particularly in analytical work.
- If you have the slightest doubt, do not proceed further. STOP, INVESTIGATE, and only then PROCEED further.

10

Mr. YASIN - SENSE OF PERSONAL RELATIONS

When one works in an industry, you work with many people at many different levels, in different work areas and with different attitudes.

On the shop floor, when you are working as a shop floor supervisor, you really work closely with the workers in your department. So closely that the positions of supervisor and workers literally get dissolved and if you really get involved with each other, then the group of workers and shop floor supervisors becomes like a small group of friends.

We had one worker by name Yasin Khan, in my section, where we used to manufacture Binaca toothpastes. Binaca-Top, Binaca-Green and Binaca-Fluoride were the top running brands of toothpastes at that time, probably next only to Colgate.

Yasin's job was to get the raw materials from the warehouse, daily, help in loading and unloading the materials from the pallets and housekeeping the toothpaste section. He might have been about thirty five years or so, and I was relatively young, in the age group of early twenties. Within a short time we developed very good relations with each other. On the shop floor we were three junior supervisors, Anil Gupte, Sharad Joshi and I.

In Binaca toothpaste section sometimes we used to work for extended hours. That meant that at 5 o'clock the general shift for the other workers used to get over, but we would continue to work upto 7 o'clock and then close the department and leave. Normally I used to go by private bus, which used to come to the gate at 5:15 P.M., but when I used to work for extended hours, I used to walk up to Kanjur Marg railway station and catch a train to Dadar and from there to Vile-Parle where I used to stay with my uncle.

We used to make two and half batches in a general shift and three batches in the extended hours. The last operation in the manufacturing used to be mixing of the toothpaste mass for 30 minutes, then closing the mixer and lastly closing the department and leaving.

Mr. Naik's strict instructions was to leave the workers at 7 o'clock sharp and the supervisor should leave at 7:30 P.M. This was to avoid an unnecessary overtime for the workers of half an hour as after 7 o'clock they did not have any work, since only the mixing was left which could be handled by the supervisor. So only one of us i.e., Anil, Sharad or I used to be there in the department between 7 to 7:30 P.M. (In fact afterwards I realised that this practise was not a good safety practice, because if something goes wrong then the only person in the department will not be able to handle it and can face serious problems. But anyway right or wrong, that was the practice at that time.)

So whenever we used to work for extended hours, Yasin always used to stay with us along with two other operators. Since we would upto 7:30 P.M., we used to feel really hungry, so we would send Yasin to a nearby hotel after 5 o'clock to get some potato vadas and bread. And then after everyone from the general shift left, we used to sit in our change room and have vada-pav. (Please don't ask me if this is in compliance with cGMP. It is not, definitely not. But at that time we were not aware of what GMP and cGMP was.)

There were some days when CIBA was going through rough industrial relations. There were problems going on with the labour unions and the management. The environment was little tense. The workers resorted to go-slow and work to rule tactics, etc. This was a typical work tactic during such unrests.

It was about 4 o'clock, Yasin called Anil and me outside the department and said, "Sir, please give me some money. I will go and get the vada-pav now itself."

"But Yasin, today we are not working extended hours, then why you need it? We are leaving at 5 o'clock itself."

"No Sir, you don't know, today exactly at 5 o'clock the labour union has planned to "Gherao" our officers and managers and I don't know how long it will continue. So I will go and get something to eat and we can have it in our change room and then even if we gherao you people and shout you will not have any problem. Also before 5 o'clock, go to the washroom and be ready for the gherao." ("Gherao" is obstructing a small group of people by a large gathering from moving from one place.")

Imagine the situation; the person who was going gherao us, himself was worried about our wellbeing. He was the most junior person in the hierarchy but with the most concern for his so called bosses. I gave him the money for the vada-pav. We ate it, went to the washroom before 5 o'clock and got ready for the gherao.

Incidentally the gherao did not last for more than an hour. Our personnel manager and Dr Patki came on the scene and the issue was resolved for the day and we went home.

After nearly forty years, I still remember the day, but more important I remember the man by name Yasin Khan, who showed unusual affection for us. He is someone that I can never forget.

I have one more story of Yasin to share with you, who demonstrated the same concern but in a different situation.

Kanjur Marg area, where our CIBA factory was situated at that time, was not a very safe locality particularly in the night. That day as usual I was working for extended hours in the department. At 7 o'clock I told Yasin to leave, I was to leave at 7:30 P.M. after the completion of final mixing and closing the department.

At 7:30, I stopped the mixer and was to put off the lights and close the department, when I found Yasin in the department. "Sir, you go and change your dress. I will close the department," he said.

"Yasin, what are you doing here till 7:30, you were supposed to leave at 7 o'clock itself," I asked him. I was thinking about tomorrow, when if I would write Yasin's leaving time as 7:30 along with mine, then Mr Naik was sure to ask me about it, and was also going to reprimand me. He was very particular about such small things.

Meanwhile Yasin told me, "Sir, you write my leaving time as 7:00 P.M. only as usual. Actually I left the factory at 7:00 P.M. only, but at the gate the security officer was telling me that there was some trouble at the station corner and even the police had become involved. Then I thought it may not be good for you to go alone from there at such a time, so I waited at the security gate till 7:30 P.M. I asked the security officer to let me come inside again and take you with me. We will go together. I could have gone alone without any problem, but you might have faced some difficulty, so I returned. Now let us go sir."

"Thank you Yasin, thank you very much"

"No Sir, you need not thank me, it was my duty."

We left the factory together. I was contemplating on what sort of man Yasin was. He might not have had access to sound education, but he was a good, affectionate and considerate person and always showed that through his behaviour. I learnt one thing from this incident, that in life, organisational positions have no relevance to one's personal behaviour.

You must have realised, why I could not forget this particular man, after more than forty years. I will probably never forget him in my entire life.

11

SKY IS THE LIMIT
(Mr. KULKARNI'S CASE)

It had not even been a month since I joined CIBA, when one day I was busy with my usual manufacturing activities and an elderly gentleman entered the department. Since he was in a white apron and a cap and looked like a senior person, I wished him.

"Good morning Sir," I said.

"Good morning," he replied. "What is your name young man?" He asked.

"I am Manohar Sir, Manohar Potdar, I am an assistant chemist here."

"Good, good, carry on."

"Yes sir" and then he left the department.

I did not dare to ask him who he was or what his name was.

"Sir, do you know who that gentleman was?" my process worker Tambade asked me.

"No I don't know. Who was he?"

"Mr. Kulkarni, the Deputy Factory Manager."

"My god! You should have told me earlier. Thank god I wished him at least," I said.

"You know sir, we used to work together," Tambade said.

"You are still working even today, is it not?" I asked.

"No Sir, not in that way. Kulkarni Sab was working with us in the tableting department as a worker, like us; and now he is the Deputy Manager."

"What are you saying Tambade? Are you mad?"

"No Sir, I am telling you the facts sir, ask Francis," he said. Farncis was one of my senior workers.

"Francis, Mr. Kulkarni Saab was working with us na? Tell Sir, he is not ready to believe it, tell him."

"Yes sir, Kulkarni Saab was a worker with us. But he was very hard working and intelligent. Once he was transferred to the tablet coating section because a worker from there, a tablet pan coater retired. From that day he learnt everything from there. Even Dalal saab or Dr. Bora used to call him to their office to consult him on any problems related to coating." Francis gave me the whole background. Dr Bora was heading the Formulation development Lab and Mr. Dalal was an F & D officer. Francis continued further, "Actually Mody Saab, our Factory Manager, wanted to make him tablet department Head, but F.D.A did not allow that since he was not qualified. So Mody Saab made him Deputy Factory Manager. Nobody objected to that, Sir."

"Thank you Francis, Thank you for giving me this information."

"Sir even today you will find him working with his own hands in the coating section, at times. Sometimes he comes to our workers canteen and takes a cup of tea with us and chats with us for some time. He is really a good man sir."

"He must be." I said.

Believe me, I never would have believed such a story if someone had told me. But since he was a live example in front of me, I could not disbelieve it. Those were the days when there were people to appreciate and respect your worth. I recollect a Hindi saying, "Hire ko pehechane ke liye johari hi chahiye."

12

MY DAYS AT PILANI

I left CIBA to take admission in Birla Institute of Technology and Science (Pilani) for doing my M. Pharm.

It was in June 1971. One of my friends, Mohan Bagade was there. He helped me in preparing for the All India Admission Test at Pilani and I finally secured admission there.

At that time there were only two specialised subjects, they were Pharmaceutical Chemistry and Pharmaceutics. I wanted pharmaceutics but got pharmaceutical chemistry. Right from the beginning I was scared of chemistry, and so I was very uncomfortable doing my M. Pharm in chemistry. I was in two minds about whether to accept the admission in pharmaceutical chemistry or go back to Mumbai and continue with my job. But my friend forced me to take admission and I did it.

Our senior batch was getting U.G.C scholarship of Rs. 250/- per month for doing M. Pharm. So we too were anticipating the same and hence were happy. But suddenly we were told that we may not get the UGC scholarship and if at all we get the scholarship then we will get it only from next semester i.e., from Jan 72.

I was once again in a dilemma. I told the admission officer, that I had to return to Mumbai to get some money and then return. He was a very nice and considerate person and gave me permission to go to

Mumbai and come back as soon as possible. He said to me, "Before you leave just meet Prof. Mittal, tell him and then leave."

I met Prof. Mittal, told him that I wanted to leave, he agreed then I left Pilani, went to Mumbai and from there to Kolhapur.

At home, there were three family members, my father, my younger sister and my younger brother.

The moment I reached home at Kolhapur, my father asked me, "What happened to your admission? Did you get in or not?"

I said, "Tatya (we used to call our father Tatya) I got the admission, but I was to get a scholarship which I am not going to get until next semester. So I think I will continue with my job instead of studying further."

"How much expenditure do you think you would incur?" he asked.

"Pilani is a little expensive. In Karad I was able to manage with hundred rupees a month but in Pilani I will need at least 200 rupees or so each month," I replied.

"That's okay, no problem. In your bank account I have deposited nearly five thousand rupees over the past two years, which you used to send me from your salary. I will send you two hundred rupees from that for your monthly expenditures," he said.

I never realised that my father had saved all the money that I sent him over the past two years.

I never said, "Thank you, Dad," but he read it in my eyes.

"Now don't waste time, get ready and rush to Pilani tomorrow itself. I will ask Nayana to do your packing. Okay?" he told me and my younger sister Nayana started packing my luggage.

A week after I was in BITS Pilani in Ram Bhavan. This was the name of the hostel at BITS, where I stayed for the next two years.

BITS Pilani was definitely a new experience to me as a student. Everything here was different compared to my old college and hostel at Karad.

In Karad three of us were staying in a single room. In BITS every student had a separate room with a ceiling fan, a table, a chair, a cot and as easy chair as well. To me it was a sort of luxury hotel. I settled into the new place shortly.

Practically every alternate week I used to send a postcard or inland letter to Kolhapur.

In Karad we used to get only lunch and dinner in the hostel, but at BITS we used to get breakfast at about 7, lunch between 12 to 1, tea and snacks at 5 P.M. and dinner at 7 to 9 P.M., all this for a fess of not more than hundred and twenty five rupees a month only. I was receiving two hundred rupees money order every month without fail. So, I was happy.

The college timing used to be 8.00 A.M. to 12 noon and from 1 P.M. to 5 P.M. in the afternoon. Saturday was a half day with college only upto 12 noon and Sunday was a holiday.

We had an auditorium-cum-cinema theatre in the college. Every semester we used to get fifteen passes to see the movies, which used to be played every Saturday and Sunday and the cost of fifteen passes used to be only fifteen rupees.

The campus of the college had a Saraswati temple and a place called Shivganga, where we used to spend some of our evenings. We also had a small market place, called Canought place, where we had two hotels, one was a very good hotel called 'Volga' and the other was a small dhaba type hotel. Volga was slightly expensive but sometimes we used to go there to eat. Paneer pakoda, vegetable biryani and coffee were the most popular dishes of the hotel. Canought place also had a grocery-cum-stationery shop and some other small shops in the market.

We also had a swimming pool in the campus, where we used to go swimming for the two years when we were at BITS.

The days were going well, but for me there was a problem. I had a gap of two years after my B.Pharm and I had really lost touch with chemistry. As such I was never interested in chemistry and the level of M. Pharm pharmaceutical chemistry was of a very high standard and I was finding it really difficult. I was not able to cope with this chemistry. Once I was sitting with a gloomy face in one corner of the room, when my friend and classmate, Debabrato Ghosh came into my room.

"Hey what happened to you? Any problem Manohar?" Deb asked me.

"Nothing yaar, nothing in particular," I replied.

"No, I don't believe you. Tell me honestly what happened? Is everything alright at home?" Deb insisted. He was really a very good friend of mine.

"Come inside, let us have a cup of tea," I invited Deb into my room, who was standing in the corridor in front of the room.

"Okay. I will make tea for you today," Deb came inside my room and started making tea. In my hostel wing, only I had arrangement for making tea.

Both of us sat on chairs with tea mugs in my hand.

"Tell me now, I am not going to leave you like that," Deb again pressed me to talk.

"Deb, I am very weak in chemistry. I am not able to cope with M. Pharm. Chemistry. Even in B. Pharm I was never comfortable with the subject. You know, in BSc., I even failed in chemistry once. I don't know what to do. I am seriously considering leaving M. Pharm and going back to Mumbai and start working again in some company," I said, opening up to Deb.

"Hey Manohar! please don't think of leaving M. Pharm and that too M. Pharm from BITS Pilani. You will never get a chance like this again. We will do something, I mean I will do something, just give me a day or two. But I am telling you, you are not going anywhere and you are going to complete your M. Pharm chemistry. I am not allowing you to do anything hasty. Is that clear?" Deb literally warned me.

My eyes were filled with tears. Deb had also become emotional.

"Hey Manohar!, don't worry yaar. Everything will be alright. We will make it alright. Relax, just relax. I will see you in the evening. Just keep in mind what I told you."

"Okay, okay, thanks Deb, thanks."

Dr. Jadav Singh was my guide. I was in the chemistry lab. I got a message saying Dr. Jadav Singh was calling me. I rushed to his room.

"May I come in Sir?"

"Yes, come, come." Dr. Singh said.

I went inside his room and stood in front of him.

"Yes Sir, you called me?"

"Sit down."

"Thank you sir," I said as I sat down on the chair.

"Deb came to me in the morning and he was talking about you."

"What, Sir?"

"He told me that you find the study of chemistry difficult and you want to leave BITS. Is it true?"

I did not say anything. There was pin drop silence. Then I slowly raised my eyes to look at him.

"Come to my house in the evening," Dr. Singh said.

"Yes sir."

"Good, go now. I will be waiting for you."

"Yes Sir."

I left his room.

At about 6 o'clock in the evening I pushed the doorbell to Singh Sir's residence. Dr. Singh's son opened the door and saw me standing there.

"Papaji, someone is here for you."

"Call him inside," Dr Singh told his son. I removed my shoes and entered the house.

"Come, come Manohar, sit down and relax." I sat down on the sofa.

"What would you like to drink, tea or coffee?" Dr. Singh asked.

"Nothing Sir, don't bother," I replied.

"Okay, we will have tea. Banti (his son) mummy ko bolna do cup chai banaye."

Dr. Singh asked for two cups of tea, placed the book on the table and relaxed a bit.

"Hmmm. Now tell me Manohar, what is the problem?"

"Sir, actually I find the study of chemistry very difficult. When I applied I was hoping to get into pharmaceutics and instead I landed up in chemistry. I requested to be transferred to pharmaceutics but Dr. Mittal said it was not possible. What to do sir?"

"Who says chemistry is difficult?"

I did not know what to answer, I just stared at him blankly.

"First of all you need to remove the fear of chemistry from your head. In fact chemistry is the simplest subject that I have ever learnt and taught."

"Sir"

"Nothing difficult. Kuch hai hi nahi isme. What difficulty do you have?"

I was silent again.

Banti brought two cups of chai for us.

"Have it," Dr. Singh offered me the tea.

"Kuch darne ka nahi samje? Pakoda khaoge?"

"No Sir, thank you. I am fine with the tea."

"But I am not, Nilu…Nilima?" Dr. Singh called for his wife.

"Ji"

"Pakoda khilaoge?"

"Ji"

"Thanks"

The meaning of Dr. Singh's request to his wife was in fact an order.

I was getting highly embarrassed. But there was no way I could avoid it.

During our discussion, with tea and pakoda, he counselled me. I really got motivated when he talked to me. The time passed very quickly and suddenly it was seven thirty. I was becoming uneasy.

"So hope you understood what I have been saying to you." Dr. Singh said.

"Yes Sir." I replied.

"By the way how much money do you have in your pocket now?" I was surprised by Dr. Singh's question. I suddenly wondered whether he wanted me to pay for the tea and pakoda. (Just joking)

I checked in my pocket and replied, "Twenty rupees Sir."

"Good, now you are going to Canaught place book stall and buy a book called Morrisson and Boyd's Organic Chemistry. It costs seventeen rupees. Do you understand?"

"Yes Sir," I said.

"I want to see that book in your hand tomorrow. Is that clear?"

"Yes Sir."

"You are going to read that book like a novel, from cover to cover. If you don't understand anything from that, ask Deb. I have already told him that he should help you with this, and if he is unable to explain it, then both of you should come to my room."

"Yes Sir."

"Finish that book in the next ten days. Okay?"

"Yes Sir."

"Remember once you have read that book, you will have no problem in understanding pharmaceutical chemistry of M. Pharm. Next ten days you are going to read only one book and that is Morrisson's chemistry. Okay?"

"Yes Sir, I will." I said.

"Good, now you can go to your hostel. And remember you are not going anywhere until you complete your M. Pharm. Understand?" Dr. Singh asked me.

"Yes Sir."

"Good."

I stood up, thanked him and left his house. Dr. Singh was really a very soft spoken person, but that day he was like an army officer and I was like a new recruit in the army.

After more than forty years now I still remember that incidence. Had Dr. Singh not called me to his house and counselled me, I probably never would have gotten my M. Pharm degree. Dr. Singh guided me for my M. Pharm thesis. When I was leaving Pilani after completing my M. Pharm, I went to his house to say I am going back to Mumbai. I bent to touch his feet; he stopped me by holding my shoulders with both his hands, looked straight into my eyes and hugged me. I could not stop my tears.

I was really lucky to have a person like Dr. Singh as my mentor, my guide; who showed me the right path by helping to develop my confidence in me. Can I ever forget a person like him in my life time?

I remember one incident, which engraved in my mind the exact and true meaning of the word "Professor".

Once, we were to have our mid-term seminar in the first week of January. All the students were to go home after the first semester exam in December and planning to come back by the end of the first week in January even though college was supposed to start from second of January.

We went to Professor Mithal and requested him to change the date of the seminar to after 8th January. But he refused bluntly and said, "No, no. The seminar will be held on the 3rd and 4th of January as the notice says."

We went to Professor Shanti Swarup Mathur, who was the most senior Professor, next only to Professor Mithal.

"Sir, can we come inside?" I asked.

"Yes, come in. What is the problem boys?" Dr. Mathur asked.

"Sir, we want your help in postponing the seminar date to second week of January Sir." I said.

"To Mithal Saab se bat karna."

"Sir, we went to Dr. Mithal, but…" Professor Mathur stopped me in between and asked, "What did you say?"

"Sir we went to Dr. Mithal" at this point he again stopped us. We were confused as to why he kept stopping us and were unable to understand how to respond. But then, Mathur sir came to our rescue.

"Never address Professor Mithal as Dr. Mithal again." Professor Mathur said.

"Anything wrong in that sir?" I asked.

"Yes, it is definitely wrong. Always address him as professor, you know he is the only professor in our department, even Dr. Banerjee and I are not professors. In our department every teacher is a doctor, but only Mittal sir is a professor. Understand?"

"Yes sir, sorry sir." I said.

What happened to our seminar date I do remember, but what I never forgot is the difference between the two words "doctor and professor."

This was the first time I realised that Professor is someone really big and great. In our Karad college, we had one doctor, he was Dr. Rashinkar, our chemistry teacher. All the others were B. Pharms and M. Pharm graduates. So we always used to call all of them professors and Dr. Rashiykar as doctor, because in our college doctor was a rare species. But in BITS Pilani practically every teacher was a doctor and professors were a rare species.

In May 1973, I finished my M. Pharm. in pharmaceutical chemistry with first class and excellent grade in my thesis. (Thanks to a guide like Dr. Jagdev Singh)

I left Pilani on 16th May 1973 with many sweet memories of those two years in mind, to come back to Mumbai, where I spent most of my life after that.

13

SWEET BENGAL BHOJAN (BITS)

Debbrato Ghosh was my classmate in M. Pharm Pilani, he was a typical Bengali babu. His English or Hindi talk always had a Bengali tinge.

It was a Saturday evening. My room in the hostel was at the end of the corridor. So on Saturdays and Sundays we used to take our chairs in the corner of the corridor and spend time drinking tea, chit chatting and eating something.

That evening Subramaniam, Paranjyoti, Dilip Kundu, and I were sitting in the corridor as usual.

"Hey what are you doing yaar?" Ghosh asked as he joined us.

"Can't you see? Come join us." Dilip replied.

"No, no I have to go to the Saraswati temple now."

"For what?" I asked.

"There is a bhojan there in the temple."

"Bhojan in the temple" I asked, my face full of surprise.

"When, when?" Subramaniam asked fully alert.

"After half an hour." Ghosh replied.

"Is it free?" Subramaniam enquired.

"Yeah, it is totally free. Anyone can join it yaar. Why don't you join me?" Ghosh invited all of us.

"I have some work, I am not coming." Dilip replied.

"Hey Deb, what will they have there in the Bhojan?" Subramaniam asked getting excited.

"This will be bengali, very sweet you know. You will enjoy it. Come, let us all go together." Ghosh insisted.

"Yaar Manohar chal yaar." Subba asked me to join. Finally we all decided to go to the temple.

"Hey Deb, why is there a bhojan today?" Paranjyoti asked inquisitively.

"Yaar Paru, why are you bothered yaar, about why and all, it is a Bengali sweet bhojan. Why should we bother about all that. Just go and enjoy the sweet Bengali bhojan and come back." Subba sealed all enquiries and we left the hostel and left for Saraswati temple.

"Yaar let us go fast otherwise it will get over." Ghosh said hurrying a little.

Finally we reached the temple at about 7 o'clock. We removed our shoes and enetered the temple.

Inside there was some Shastri ji singing some prayer and two other persons were accompanying him on the tabla (drum) and the harmonium.

Ghosh asked us to be seated beside some other Bengali people. Subba and I went and sat together.

"Yaar Manohar, where is the bhojan.?"

"It will be arranged somewhere nearby. Why?"

"When yaar? I am hungry." Subba said a little uneasily.

"I think the bhojan will be after this prayer song." I said trying to calm him down.

"Yaar we should have come a little late. I don't know when this prayer song will get over. Did we come for this or for the bhojan?"

"Okay. Have some patience yaar. Once this is over we will have bhojan yaar." I stopped Subba's further enquiries.

The prayer song business went on till eight in the night.

"Hey Manu let us go." Deb said.

Everyone from our group got up and came out of the temple.

"How was the bhojan? Did you like it?" Deb asked.

"Where was the bhojan?" Subbu almost screamed.

"What do you mean Subbu? What do you mean by where is the bhojan?" Ghosh asked completely puzzled. "What the hell were you listening to for the last one hour?"

"What? That is the bhojan that you were talking about, Deb?" Subba asked totally annoyed.

"Yeah. What else? Did you not like it Subba?"

"But you said Bhojan. This was some prayer song."

"Yeah, this is what we called bhojan."

"But you were talking about Bengali sweet bhojan."

"Yeah it was Bengali only and I thought it was very sweet. Did you not like it?" Ghosh was trying to explain this Bengali sweet bhojan to Subbu.

"You rascal, we thought we were going for Bengali sweet dinner."

"I never said that, did I, Manu?" Ghosh came to me for rescue.

Ghosh got really scared. Subbu was twice his size.

"Subba wait let me explain things." I intervened.

"Subba, when Ghosh talked about "bhojan" he meant "bhajan" i.e., songs of god, or rather sweet songs of god in Bengali language. And all of us understood "bhojan" as dinner, and that too with Bengali sweets like, rasagolla, sandesh and all." I replied.

"Oh my god, this Bengali fellow, does not know how to pronounce bhajan. I will beat you, you rascal." Subha was really annoyed.

"Okay. Yaar Subba it is not his fault. It is ours too." I said trying to calm Subba down.

Finally it was settled that Ghosh will give us all a treat at Nutan market. Everybody later laughed at the funny incident, and Subba enjoyed the treat given by Ghosh and even asked, "So Deb, when are you giving the next bhojan?" and to this Ghosh replied, "Even if I know, I will never tell you people."

We thoroughly enjoyed the treat given by Ghosh, even though it was not the "Sweet Benagli Bhojan" that we were looking forward to.

14

LAST DAY IN BITS PILANI

We were only three students in chemistry in our batch in M. Pharm. Mr. Ghosh, Mr. Kundu and I.

It was the last day in the college, next day all of us were to leave our beloved BITS. Dr Rajdhan sent a message to all of us to meet him in his room.

Dr. Rajdhan used to teach us synthetic chemistry and chemistry practical too of the first year.

We were not aware as to why he had called us. Kundu said it was probably because there was some problem with the returning of the glassware or some such thing.

We entered his room and all greeted him in unison, "Good morning Sir." He slowly raised his head, removed his spectacles, placed them on the table, rubbed his face slightly with his palms and paused for a moment. We looked at each other. The room suddenly became slightly tense.

"So today is your last day here, is it?"

"Yes sir."

"How is the lab?"

"Good sir."

"Good means?"

"Good means good. Okay Sir."

"What okay?"

"The lab sir."

"I know that." We were getting slightly scared.

"Sit down." He ordered.

We sat down in the chairs in front of Dr. Rajdhan.

"I want the lab as it was when you first entered it." Dr. Rajdhan demanded. We looked at each other and Kundu had a slightly mischievous look on his face.

"Okay sir." I said.

"Now you may go and get the lab key to me in the afternoon. Okay?"

"Yes sir," we replied and left the room.

We went to the lab. It was perfectly alright. Everything was in place. We even called the lab peon and asked him to just get it cleaned once again.

When we had come to BITS two years back, Dr. Mittal had told us that there is a separate small room in front of Dr. Rajdhan's room, you get that room cleaned, and organise your lab there, that is a nice place. You three can work there in that lab for the next two years. We were very happy because the room was at one corner of the department. The only problem was that Dr. Rajdhan used to sit in front of that lab.

When we opened the room, we got the shock of our lives. The room was a total mess, probably not used for months. It was all dirty. We called the peon and all of us together began to clean the room. Dilip Kundu found two dead rats in the room. He threw them away. It took nearly two days to clean the room and then another week to make it look like a chemistry lab. Luckily water, light and gas connections were already there.

Finally after one week we started working in the lab. This was the story of the lab two years back. In the afternoon at about three, we went to Dr. Rajdhan.

"Good afternoon sir." We said.

"Good afternoon. Is the lab okay?"

Dilip Kundu was a mischievous fellow. Secondly he was there for the last six years in BITS. So he was more familiar with the institute and the teachers also.

"Sir, there is a little problem." Dilip started.

"What problem?"

"Sir you wanted us to leave the lab as we found it when we first entered it." Dilip continued.

"Any issue? Any problem?"

"Yes sir." Dilip replied.

"Yes sir. What do you mean?"

"Sir outside the building there is sufficient sand, available but we could get the dead rats Sir." Dilip said and annoyed Dr. Rajdhan.

"What nonsense, why do you need the dead rats?" Dr. Rajdhan said in an annoyed voice.

"No sir, Dilip is just playing a joke. Since on the first day when we entered the lab, two years ago, it was full of dirt, sand and we also found two dead rats at that time. But now the lab is perfectly okay sir. Don't worry sir." I said trying to calm down Dr. Rajdhan.

"You Dilip................." Dr. Rajdhan was going to say something in an annoyed voice.

Ghosh intervened, "Sir today is our last day sir." Hearing this Dr. Rajdhan calmed down.

"Sir, here are the keys, I am sorry sir." Dilip apologised and handed over the keys to Dr. Rajdhan.

Dr. Rajdhan looked at us; all of our faces were gloomy. Dr. Rajdhan got up from his chair and came in front of the table towards us. He looked at us again.

"Smile yaar, smile." Dr. Rajdhan extended both his hands towards us. We held his hands and then later touched his feet.

"We will miss you sir, we will never forget you." We said wiping our wet eyes.

"I too will miss you, take care."

"Thank you sir, thank you very much." We said and then left his room.

15

TURNING POINT

From Pilani I came straight to Kolhapur, my native place. I thought I spend some time relaxing with my family and my friends, because I was away from home for nearly two years, except for short vacations in December and May.

Somewhere in mid June 1973 I came to Mumbai in search of a job. The period was not so good. After B. Pharm I got a job within a months' time, but after M. Pharm, for nearly five months I was jobless. Finally I got frustrated and wrote a letter to Professor Mittal asking if he could give me a job, I would like to come back to Pilani. To my great surprise within 15 days I got his reply. I received a letter mentioning that BITS has offered me a job of Assistant lecturer and the salary will be nine hundred and sixty rupees and will be given a staff quarters for ninety six rupees a month plus I can avail the facility of the hostel mess for breakfast, lunch and dinner. I was really very happy.

I talked to my father about this job. His comments were a little cautious, he said "If you are not getting a job in Mumbai then you can go there, but if you get a job in Mumbai, you take that job instead of going all the way to Pilani again."

I really had no choice. I convinced my father and planned to leave to Pilani, and booked a ticket up to 'Chirava'.

My friend Mohan Bagade was working in Sarabhai chemicals in Baroda. I was always in touch with him. I told him that I am planning to go back to Pilani, I confirmed the date and time of my train journey to him. I was going to travel by Paschim express, which used to reach Baroda in the evening of the same day. I asked him to see me at the platform at Baroda.

The train reached Baroda at about 6 o' clock in the evening. Mohan was already on the platform, we met and he forced me to take a break of one day and stay back at Baroda. A friend of his was a T.C and he managed to get my break journey approved by him. I also got the reservations for the next day.

I got down and went to Mohan's room where he was staying as a bachelor along with one of his friends, who was also working in Sarabhai chemicals.

We spent that evening moving around the city, had dinner in a good vegetarian restaurant and came back to the room and took rest.

The next day my train was in the evening. Mohan suggested that I accompany him to his factory in the morning. Since I had no other work I decided to accompany him. When we reached the factory, we came to know that there were some interviews arranged for that day for the job of Q.C Chemist. Mohan introduced me to Ms Desai who was the Personnel Manager there. She suggested that I should appear for the interview and I agreed.

From there onwards the things went very smoothly, after nearly five months of waiting. I appeared for the interview and got selected along with another friend from BITS, V.S. Subramaniam. Only two of us, out of nearly twenty candidates got selected. Now the big question was what to do. Should I go to back to BITS or should I join Sarabhai chemicals? Subramaniam, Mohan and Ms Desai insisted that I should join Sarabhai chemicals. I sent a telegram communicating my inability to come to BITS Pilani to Dr Mithal, and I joined Sarabhai chemicals and not BITS Pilani.

This moment changed my life altogether I became an industrial pharmacist instead of becoming a teacher at a university. I continued my industrial life from that day until 30th June 2005, a long span of nearly 32 years.

From now onwards I am going to talk about my life as an industrial pharmacist.

Remember this is not really my autobiography, even though at times it may sound like one, but the narration of some selected incidents in this long period of 32 years and also another seven years as a university teacher, from February 2006 till October 2012.

This is a long journey and I am going to take you with me, showing and telling you on the way what I faced and how I enjoyed myself and the lessons I learnt and the blunders I committed and much more.

Some of the incidents are serious and others are funny; these I call the 'lighter side of life'. You will meet so many people, right from operators and workers to plant heads and Managing Directors, FDA officials, IAS officers, many government officials, some good and some not so good. You are going to meet even some unusual political leaders; some people who believed in the "call beyond the duty", some friends who helped me without expecting anything in return and also some "friends" who never thought beyond themselves.

When you read this book, if you are an industrial pharmacist already, you will be able to identify with this story and you will find that many incidences are similar to what you are experiencing or have experienced. If you are a student and are thinking of selecting a career as an industrial pharmacist, you will know what the life of an industrial pharmacist involves, what mistakes can happen, what mistakes I made and hence you can avoid making those mistakes in your own career.

I assure you this is going to be an interesting read for all pharmacists, both for those who are already in the industry and for those who will soon join the industry. This will be a very good companion reader for pharmacy students along with their study of pharmacy.

Am I making sense? Are you ready for the journey? Yes?

Good! Then let's go.

16

MY FIRST JOB AFTER M. PHARM

In fact my first job after M. Pharm was with Sarabhai chemicals, Baroda, but I do not refer to that as my first job, since I worked there for a very short span of time, less than two months. Hence what is in reality my second job; I call as my first job, as I stayed on with that job for more than seven years or so.

I had continued living with Mohan since his second room partner did not mind, the room was big enough to easily accommodate all three of us and best of all was that the three of us were very compatible with each other and enjoyed living together.

Mohan and I reached the room at about 5:30 P.M. Pradeep our third room partner was already in the room, since he had not gone to work because he was unwell. The moment we entered the room Pradeep said, "Manohar, there is a letter here for you from Hoechst."

"Hoechst?" I asked in surprise, "Show me." I was excited about it. I opened the letter and got shocked. It was a call for an interview in response to one of my applications for a job which I had sent nearly four months back, when I was in Mumbai, which was redirected to me by my uncle.

I read it carefully. The interview was on next Monday and today was Thursday, that meant that I had minimum two days in hand. I had to leave to Mumbai either on Saturday or Sunday. I thought of leaving on Saturday evening itself so that I would arrive in Mumbai one day prior to the interview.

Getting leave on Monday was just not possible since I had not even completed two months at the job. We sat together and discussed what I should do. Pradeep said, " Manohar don't tell anything to Ambubhai (who was my boss), you leave without informing him. On Monday I will tell him that your uncle was not well and so you had to leave suddenly and go to Mumbai." All of us agreed on this plan of action.

The interview was for production pharmacist and I was working in Q.C. Of course earlier I had worked in CIBA as a production pharmacist for some time, so I did have some exposure. Next two days Mohan, Pradeep and I discussed the many different aspects of production during the evenings, in preparation to face the interview on Monday.

Saturday evening I left Baroda to go to Mumbai.

It was a cool Monday morning of December 1973 in Mumbai. I entered the posh reception hall of Hoechst India Ltd. a German multinational pharmaceutical company in Mulund-Mumbai.

A young and smart receptionist was sitting in the reception office. I went up to her and greeted her.

"Good morning Ma'am."

"Good morning," She replied with a sweet smile.

"I am Potdar, Manohar Potdar. I have an interview for the post of Production chemist." At that time even for the job of a pharmacist, the word pharmacist was not very popular, it was called chemist. "Yes, I have the list with me; there are three other candidates who were being also interviewed for the post. They will be arriving shortly. The interviews will start at 10:30, you may please take a seat over there."

"Thank you ma'am," I said. I looked at my wristwatch. It was 10:05 and there was still about half an hour to go before the interview. When I heard there were three other candidates appearing for the interview, my confidence was a little shaken and I became a little uneasy. I sat on the sofa at the reception for a while, got up again and moved to the main door, looked outside and came back and sat on the sofa again.

The receptionist probably sensed my uneasiness and asked, "Mr. Potdar, would you like a glass of water?"

"No, it's okay, thank you." I replied.

"Relax man, relax, there is still half an hour left," she pushed a bell somewhere and a boy came to her. "Raghu, can you get Mr. Potdar a glass of water," she said to him.

Raghu went to get a glass of water; I sat down on the sofa again and started looking at my file.

"Hey Manohar!, what are you doing here man?"

I looked up in surprise. My classmate from Karad, Shrikar Kulkarni was standing in front of me in a white apron, with a cap on his head.

"Hey! How come you are here?" I asked in surprise.

"I am working with Hoechst for the last two years."

"What a great surprise, I have an interview today at 10:30 here."

"Good yaar," he said as he sat down beside me.

"What will they ask me in the interview? I am quite scared actually."

"Don't worry Manohar. But keep in mind that our Technical Director, Dr Habischt, has a habit of asking any type of question, may not necessarily be related to pharmacy. But you don't worry. All the best. I have to go back inside now. I'll see you soon," Shrikar said as he left. Then suddenly he returned and said, "Manohar ask for a salary of a thousand rupees. Okay?" he said and left.

Raghu got me a glass of water, I thanked him.

The main door opened and I saw two more candidates entering. Looking at their appearance I felt that I had a good chance of getting selected. I relaxed a little bit.

"Mr. Potdar, can I have your letter please?" the receptionist asked for my interview call letter. I got up and handed her the letter.

"Just wait for five minutes, you will be called for the interview, proceed through the door on the left and go into the last conference room." She said.

"But not immediately, I will tell you when to go. Till such time you can wait here. Okay?"

"Yes ma'am." I replied.

Meanwhile one more candidate entered the hall. I was mentally preparing myself for the interview.

"Mr. Potdar, you can go in, best of luck." the receptionist said.

"Thank you ma'am." I said and entered through the door on the left of the reception hall and started walking. Raghu was there in the corridor, he opened the conference door and I entered inside.

The room was quite big, with an oval table inside and a big office chair, on which an elderly, white, smart looking man was sitting there all dressed in white. Beside him, there was a senior Indian person, also wearing a white dress, and to his side there was another gentleman with full beard and bald head.

The bearded person welcomed me, "Come in Mr. Potdar, I am Mr. George Menezes, Personnel Manager," He introduced himself.

"Hello," I replied.

"Meet Dr. Habischt and Dr. Ravi Rosha," he introduced the other two gentlemen, "Dr. Habischt is the Technical Director and Dr. Rosha is our Manufacturing Head."

I said hello to them both.

"Take your seat Mr. Potdar." Dr. Rosha said.

"Dr. Habischt, Mr. Potdar has done his M. Pharm from BITS Pilani this year, before that he also had two years of experience with MSD and CIBA." Mr. Menezes introduced me to Dr. Habischt.

"Good." Dr. Habischt nodded his head in appreciation.

Then some introductory questions were asked by Dr. Ravi Rosha, which I answered quite satisfactorily. "Tell me, Mr. Potdar, what are the things that are required to make a good table?" Dr. Habischt asked in a typical German accent.

I suddenly remembered what Shrikar had told me, that Dr. Habischt had a habit of asking any question, not necessarily related to pharmacy.

In a small span of time I had mentally prepared myself to answer this question. In my mind I had arranged the answer as; first you will need good quality wood, probably a teak wood, then wood polish, screws, etc.

I started, "Sir, first of all we will need very good quality woo…d."

Mr. Menezes realised what a blunder I was going to make and came to my rescue by saying, "Mr. Potdar, Mr. Habischt wants to know what the requirements are to make a good TABLET….tablet." He stressed on the word tablet.

"Yes, yes we require good quality active ingredients, expeints,….blah…blah…," I said trying to salvage the situation.

"Okay, okay. Good, good." Dr. Habischt said.

"Any more questions sir?" Dr. Rosha asked Dr. Habischt.

"No, no." Dr. Habischt said.

"Thank you Mr. Potdar, you can go wait in the reception hall for some time." Mr. Menezes said to me.

I profusely thanked all of them and left the room.

I got the job and joined Hoechst India on 21st December, 1973.

I have never forgotten this interview, I do not know what would have happened if I had continue to talk about the requirements for making a table instead of a tablet. Thanks to Mr. George Menezes for his timely interruption and saving the situation.

After the interview was over, I was called to the personnel manager's office. Mr. Bhende was probably the manager next to Dr. Menezes. He called me in, "Sit down Mr. Potdar."

I sat down.

"Good news for you, you are selected, you got the job. There are just a few formalities that are to be completed before joining. Tell me, what are your expectations in terms of salary?"

I remembered Shrikar again, he had said to ask for a thousand rupees, but I was scared to ask for so much since in Sarabhai I was earning only five hundred rupees, but finally I gathered my courage and said, "Seven hundred and fifty sir."

"Seven fifty?" I could not read Mr. Bhende's expression as he said this.

"Okay……….Okay," Bhende said. "The medical officer will be coming at 12:30, you will see him there, he sits in our medical room, Liz will show you. You finish the medical check- up and come back and see me here again. Okay?"

"Yes sir."

"Liz, please take Mr. Potdar to our medical room, take these papers also and give them to Dr. D'souza's assistant." Bhende told Liz, probably his secretary I guessed.

Dr. D'souza, a medical doctor, looked like a typical Goan with a French cut beard. He examined me; he was quite an elderly person. He put my papers in an envelope and handed them over to me.

"Carry these to Mr. Bhende, god bless you." said Dr. D'souza.

I thanked him and left his office.

It was 1:30 P.M. when I entered Mr. Bhende's office; he was just leaving for lunch.

"Oh you finished the medical is it?"

"Yes sir, Dr. D'souza asked me to hand you this envelope." I said as I handed over the envelope to him.

He opened the envelope, had a cursory look at it and said, "Good, everything is okay. Shall we meet after lunch? Or are you in a hurry?"

"No sir, as you wish." I said.

"Okay, come inside and sit down." I sat down in the chair in front of him.

"When can you join Mr. Potdar?" Mr. Bhende asked.

"Sir, I was thinking I will go home and then come back and join on the 2nd of January sir." I replied.

"2 Jan? No, no, no, no, that is not acceptable. You have to join before December 23rd not later than that." He read the reluctance on my face, to join immediately. And I could see in his face the hint of a smile which he was trying to hide. "Okay sir. I will join on December 23rd." my voice clearly showing my reluctance. "You can join even before that if you want to." He looked straight into my eyes and said.

"Okay sir. I will try." I said.

"That's good. That's like a man." He called Liz and said, "Liz take him to lunch with you and then come back to the office and type his offer letter in form no. 32, meanwhile I too will have lunch and come back."

"Okay sir," Liz told him.

I had my lunch and then received my offer letter. I thanked Mr. Bhende and also did not forget to thank Liz, and lastly on the way back I also thanked the receptionist, Mary Sequera.

17

MY FIRST DAY AT HOECHST

My career with Hoechst started on 23rd December 1973. I stayed there for nearly 7 years and I learnt a lot during those 7 years of my stay in the company. The environment at Hoechst was very congenial. The management had a pro-employee attitude. I met many people who became my life-long friends. All my days at Hoechst were memorable.

On the morning of 23rd December I was waiting in the reception. It was my first day in Hoechst.

"Mr. Potdar, you go to the second floor in production, and meet Mr. Kanetkar, he is the head of the injectable department, you will be working in that department. Okay?" Mary told me. I then left for the second floor to meet Mr. Kanetkar.

Kanetkar was a very elderly looking, half-bald person. He was sitting in a small room. "Good morning sir. I am Potdar, Manohar Potdar." He raised his head and looked at me but did not move an inch from the chair.

"Wait" was the single word response from him. My first impression about my boss was not so good. I waited.

"Rajani, call Jaisingh." Kanetkar called a girl by name Rajani.

"Yes sir," Rajani said and went to call Jaisingh.

I was standing there uncomfortably. Meanwhile a young man in a white boiler suit came, I guessed that he was probably Jaisingh. My guess turned out to be right.

"Jaisingh, ye tumhare naye sahib hai, inko under leke jao aur sab dikhana, thik se."

"Ji sir."

I went with Jaisingh. "What is the meaning of inside Jaisingh?" I asked.

"Inside means in the sterile filling area sir, please come with me. I will take you, don't worry, I will show you everything." Jaisingh comforted me.

I entered the first vestibule (1st room of the change room). He showed me how to change from civil dress, where to keep it, how to wear the one piece boiler suit, how to wear nose mask, head gear, over shoes, etc. it was my first experience and it was quite tough. But Jaisingh was a very decent and sober person. He was very patient and he guided me properly.

"Sir you may find it a little difficult initially, but don't worry, it is very easy and you will get accustomed to it." Jaisingh said to me, while I was changing my dress.

Finally we went inside, Jaisingh showed me the filtration unit, the vial and ampoule filling machines. He then introduced me to some operators by name, "Sir she is Kamal, and that girl is Laxmi and the one you met in the filtration unit was Mithilda" All the girls were in full closed uniform. I could not recognise anyone; however I just nodded my head with a smile on my face inside my head gear. I could only recognise Jaisingh because of his tall figure. He took me to lunch with him. I was with him till 4 o'clock that day.

At 4 o'clock Mr. Kanetkar called me to his office, and asked me,

"Yes, Manohar, how was your first day?"

"Good sir, it was really good."

"That is fine. Tomorrow you can come in the morning at 7 o'clock, the bus starts from Mulund west. Once you arrive assemble the 3 stroke-strunk ampoule filling machine, keep it ready so that the operators who come in the morning at 8 o'clock will be able to start the filling the ampoules without any delay. Okay?"

"Okay sir."

"Any questions?"

"No sir"

You can imagine, it was just the first day in this company and in this department, and the boss was telling me to assemble the strunk-3stroke ampoule filling machine and keep it ready. I was one hundred per cent sure, that I would not be able to do the work, but I was still damn scared to say that. I just said okay for everything. I thought in my mind that I was making the biggest blunder of my life by saying "okay sir" since I had no choice.

I went back to the department and talked to Jaisingh about this. He said, "There is nothing difficult, you should be able to do it. Sir." I could not see any solution to the problem. I tried to collect as much information as possible and left the department with a lot of puzzles in my mind.

I reached Mulund west at sharp 6:30 A.M. I was not even aware where the bus stop was. To my rescue I found a tea stall (Tapari) open and a few people having tea there.

"Excuse me, can you tell me where the Hoechst bus stops?" I asked the tea stall man.

"Here itself. It will come at any moment now. Till then, would you like to have a cup of tea sir?"

"Yes, give me one."

I had a hot cup of tea and paid the money and then I saw the bus coming.

"Sir, this is the bus, you can catch that."

"Thank you, thank you very much." I thanked the tea-man and caught the bus.

There were only a few people in the bus, no one I knew. Nobody knew me. I was a little scared. It took about fifteen minutes to reach the factory from there.

I got down along with the others. I was totally unaware of how to proceed. I was just standing there; one boy came up to me and asked me, "Sir, where do you want to go?"

"Ampoule department," I said.

"Are you new?"

"Yes."

"Sir, the keys will be at the security office, come with me I will show you."

"Thanks, please show me."

He came with me and led me to the security office, where a security guard was sitting.

"Ranaji inko ampoule ki chabi dena, naye saab hai," he said to the security guard.

"Okay, okay."

The guard handed over a bunch of keys to me and asked me to enter the details in a register. I did that. The boy was still standing there.

"Sir, can I go?" he asked me.

"Yes, thank you, by the way what is your good name?" I asked.

"Chatar Singh, I work in the ointment department as an operator. Can I go now?" he asked me.

"Yes, thanks again Chatar Singh." I thanked him and started climbing the stairs to the second floor.

I had a bunch of keys with at least seven or eight keys in it. It was a great problem to find out which key fit the first vestibule, from where I was supposed to go inside.

I was struggling with the keys and the lock, I heard somebody who said, "Sir give it to me, I will open it."

I looked back and saw Jaisingh.

"Hey Jaisingh. How come you are here so early in the morning?"

"Kanetkar sab asked me to come and help you sir." He took the keys from me and opened the door, "Sir, number twenty seven key is for this door." Jaisingh told me.

"Oh okay. Thank you."

I suddenly found myself very comfortable in his presence.

"Jaisingh, when did Kanetkar sab talk to you?" I asked.

"Immediately after he spoke to you sir."

"What did he say?"

"He said, 'Potdar naya hai, usko kuch aata jaata nahi, machine tod dega.' Please help him."

"Anything else?"

"He said, 'Jaisingh, don't assemble the machine, just show him how to do it and let him assemble it. I want him to learn everything."

"Okay."

When I passed out from BITS Pilani I was really proud about myself, that I hold an M. Pharm degree from BITS Pilani, that too in first class with an 'Excellent grade' in thesis. I studied under eminent teachers like Professor B.M. Mithal, S.S. Mathur, S.K. Banerjee. Dr. Jagadev Singh was my guide and there were so many other things I was proud of. No doubt the school was very good, the teachers were well known and the degree had a great value, but even so I was still lacking something, "Practical experience." Jaisingh, an eight standard passed, skilled machine operator was my first guru in the industry, who taught me how to wear sterile garments, how to tie the overshoes, how to assemble a 3-stroke ampoule filling machine, how to assemble a filtration unit, even how to adjust ampoule sealing flame of the machine and many more things, which no college teacher teach or books like Leon Lachman or Avis ever writes about. This can be learnt only by practice and only from highly skilled operators like Jaisingh. Why do I still remember Jaisingh? It is both for his skill and his wonderful helpful attitude he showed towards me and towards many more people like me.

18

PRO-EMPLOYEE ATTITUDE

On 24th afternoon, Mr. Bhende, our assistant personnel manager called me to his office.

"How are you Mr. Potdar? Are you okay with the working environment here? Getting settled in?" he asked.

"Yes sir. I am doing very well and getting settled in. Life is tough but the people are good."

"From tomorrow i.e., December 25th till 1st January we are closed for Christmas. Now you can go to Kolhapur to meet your father. You wanted to go na?"

"Yes sir, Thank you sir," I thanked him and left his office.

A few things that I highly appreciate about this company Hoechst.

The company had a pro-employee attitude, which was not verbalized but demonstrated by the managers like, George Menezes, by saving the situation, when in the interview I misunderstood Dr Habischt question as table instead of tablet. Mr. Bhende who forced me to join on the 23rd even though he knew I wanted to go home and anyway I was to get a holiday from December 25th to January 1st. He could have easily accepted my request to join from January 2nd, 1974, but he did not do so. I realised why he did that only four months later. I received my first increment after only three months i.e. on April 1st, 1974. The company rule was that any employee who joins before December 31st of any year is entitled for his first increment on 1st

April. Had I joined on 2nd January 1974, I would have only gotten a promotion on April 1st, 1975 i.e., after fifteen months. One may not feel the importance of that after forty years, but at that time it felt great.

I asked for a salary of seven hundred and fifty per month, but when I received my first salary slip it said eight hundred and fifty. I asked Mr. Bhende if something was wrong. He said no, our starting salary for M. Pharm was eight hundred and fifty only.

When Mr Kanetkar asked me on my very first day at the job, to come the next day and assemble the ampoule filling machine. I thought in my mind what type of boss is he? Could he not realise that I may not be able to do this task. But I was wrong Kanetkar definitely knew what my capabilities were, but did not say anything to me, instead he just sent someone to help me without my knowledge, because he wanted me to develop the necessary skill and also the confidence. This was really great of Mr. Kanetkar.

Things were going smoothly. I was transferred to the sterile ointment section. I remember a few incidents that are worth mentioning.

19

BIG BAG SMALL BAG INCIDENT

We used to manufacture an ointment called 'Jadit-H' containing buclosamide and hydrocortisone. For a batch of 200 kg we used to add 20 kg of buclosamide and 1.1 kg of hydrocortisone. Hydrocortisone always used to come as one sealed bag of one kg and 100 gm in a small plastic bag. The store keeper always used to keep that small bag of 100 gm at the bottom of the container and above that the sealed 1.0 kg bag of hydrocortisone.

Chater Singh was the regular operator who used to take the batches of ointment including Jadit-H.

The bulk batch used be ready by about 3:00 P.M. and Lata, the regular Q.C. chemist used to analyse the sample of hydrocortisone. Next day morning I used to ask Lata, if the assay was okay and once it was ready, I used to start filling the batch.

Our ointment department and Q.C. lab were opposite each other of the mid-way corridor.

One day Chater Singh, my regular operator, was absent and I had to take a substitute operator. The substitute was Rajayya, who was not very familiar with the process, but at the same time he was not a totally new operator. He used to sometimes help Chater Singh.

I started the melting operation of the ointment base, filtered it hot and transferred it to the main mixer and started the stirrer at a slow speed and started circulating cool water in the jacket for cooling the base. The base has to come to about 50 degree centigrade. Then we have to add the buclosamide and then hydrocortisone and continue stirring till it is thoroughly mixed. Then the inbuilt homogeniser should be run for fifteen minutes and then the operation stops.

I explained everything to Rajayya and I said, you do what I have explained and in the meanwhile I will go to the canteen, have a cup of tea and come back, then you can go for tea. This was our regular practice, so that there is always someone in the department at all times. Rajayya was a very sincere worker.

When I came back I asked him, "Rajayya, how far have you come in the process?"

He said, "Sir, the temperature was less than fifty degrees, I have added all the ingredients and mixed them. You just have to homogenise it."

"Have you added both the bags?" I asked. I wanted to confirm that he had added both the bags of hydrocortisone: the 1 kg bag and the 100 gm bag.

"Yes sir, I added both the bags."

"Good now you can go have tea and come back, then we will go and unload the batch."

"Okay Sir, I will be back in five minutes sir."

"Okay, okay" I said as Rajayya left for the canteen.

(Now please don't ask me, what happened to that cGMP rule of "Added by, Checked by". The material was added by Rajayya and was supposed to be checked by me but was not checked. I am sorry, but it was way back in 1975.)

Next day in the morning as usual I asked Lata about the assay of hydrocortisone, she said it was okay, and I went ahead with the next step of ointment preparation, that is loading the ointment into the filling hopper. Pushpa Kadam was the machine operator who was supposed to start the tube filling operation. Everything was okay till then.

Suddenly my regular operator Chatar Singh, who was present on that day, came running towards me and said, "Sir ask Pushpa not to start the batch filling operation."

"Why? What happened?" I asked.

"Sir I think there is some problem with the batch."

"Tell me what the problem is. Don't confuse me." I said sounding a little annoyed.

"Sir who added the hydrocortisone yesterday?"

"Rajayya."

"Probably he added only one bag, it appears that he didn't add the other bag, i.e. the 100 gm bag."

"What?" I shouted.

"Yes sir. That 100 gm bag is still intact at the bottom of this container. I wanted to go through the empty container but I saw the 100 gm bag with the material inside."

I immediately asked Pushpa to stop the filling. Luckily the filling had not yet started till then.

"Okay okay Chatar Singh. I am just coming." I said as I ran to the Q.C lab.

"Lata, was the hydrocortisone assay okay yesterday?"

"Why? Why are you asking this question?" Lata asked a little worried.

"Lata, I think I have added less hydro in the batch."

Meanwhile Mohan Kumar, our assistant Q.C. manager appeared on the scene.

"Hey, what's wrong Lata? Manohar, what happened?"

I explained to him what had happened.

"Lata, do you have the sample?"

"Yes"

"Analyse it again immediately."

"Mohan, I think we should take a fresh sample from the batch, what do you say?" I asked.

"Yeah."

We analysed a fresh sample. The assay of hydrocortisone was about 91%.

"How come you said it was okay Lata?" Mohan asked.

"Actually sir the assay was coming less only but it never happened in the past so I thought there must be something wrong with the analysis and Manohar wanted to start the filling, so I said you go ahead, I was to reanalyse it, but meanwhile he came and asked about the assay. I am sorry sir." Lata was in tears.

"Manohar, how did you add less?" Mohan asked me.

I narrated the story to him.

"Now please go and add the required quantity yourself, mix it, homogenise it and then tell me, I will come myself and collect the sample and till I give you clearance do not proceed with the filling Okay?"

"Yes sir." I said.

Afterwards I called Rajayya and asked, "Rajayya, you said you added both bags, but it seems you added only one bag."

"No sir, I added both the bags."

We were still puzzled.

"Are you sure you added both the bags? One bag is big and the other is small."

"Yes sir, by god, I swear I added them both."

"Rajayya, show me which two bags you added?"

"That one big bag, you can ask Pushpa, she helped me lift that bag for adding in the mixer."

"What? You need Pushpa to help you lift the 1 kg bag?" Rajayya are you mad?" I was getting angry.

"One kg bag sir? I added only that small bag sir. Pushpa helped me to add the big bag." Rajayya was still confirming.

Meanwhile Chatar Singh started laughing.

"Chatar Singh, will you please stop laughing. You don't understand the seriousness of the situation at all." I scolded Chatar Singh.

"Sir, I understand what has happened." Chatar Singh said.

"What, what happened? Tell me."

"I will tell you sir, there is a small confusion between the 'big bag' and the 'small bag'. You are talking about the 'Big bag' of hydrocortisone and the 'small bag' of 100 gm of hydrocortisone."

"Of course."

"But Rajayya is talking about the 'big bag' of 20 kg of Buclosamide and the 'small bag' is the 1 kg bag of hydrocortisone. He is probably not even aware that there is a smaller 100 gm bag of hydrocortisone in the same container in which the bigger bag of hydrocortisone is kept."

"My God!" the whole puzzle of the big and small bag was finally solved. I too laughed.

"What happened sir, why are you both laughing." Rajayya asked very innocently.

"Chatar Singh, tell him." I told Chatar Singh and left the scene.

Since I am not going to teach cGMP here, I am not analysing the case further. You know where we should be worrying about, and what you should avoid. Remember this is year 2013 and not 1975. In the last 38 years everything has changed.

20

MID NIGHT WALK - A MATTER OF ATTITUDE

As you know, I started working with injectable department in Hoechst. We were three pharmacists in the department other than Mr. Kanetkar who was our boss.

In the morning shift there used to be three pharmacists, two of us and Mr. Kanetkar himself. In the second shift there used to be only one pharmacist.

I was the most junior pharmacist in the department, and so I used to come every alternate week in the second shift.

The last activity in the second shift used to be completing the sterilisation cycle for the change parts for the next day's morning shift, since we used to use the same parts for filling. The last sterilisation cycle had to get over before I could leave the department. The second shift bus used to leave at 11:20 P.M. sharp. That meant that I had to leave the department by 11:05 latest.

Many a times if the filling of the ampoules gets delayed, then the sterilisation cycle used to get late, and I had no choice but to wait till the sterilisation cycle gets over, in which case I would definitely miss the bus. Out of five days in a week, I used to miss the bus at least twice and sometimes more.

There was no harm in getting late by 15-20 minutes but missing the company bus had serious consequences.

The first thing was I had to take a mid-night walk from our factory to Mulund station. That was about a fifty minutes' walk on a lonely road. Secondly, I never used to be sure when I would get the train after mid night. Sometimes I had to wait for one to one and half hours and I would reach home at about 2:30-3:00 A.M. This midnight walk was really annoying, but I had no choice.

I had a very good friend in the company, in my department itself. Once I told this to him,

"Yaar Dinkar (name is changed for obvious reasons) I am really getting annoyed because I keep missing the bus. It is really horrible." I said.

"Why? Why do you miss the bus?" he questioned.

"I miss the bus because I usually get delayed by about 15-20 minutes. The last sterilisation cycle gets slightly delayed if the filling gets delayed even for ten minutes."

"Are you mad? I never miss my bus."

"How do you manage that every day?"

"I close the filling department right in time."

"Filling never gets delayed, even a single day?" I asked in surprise.

"Look, there are some manufacturing tricks. You should know them."

"What tricks?" I asked very innocently.

"See, in my shift also the filling gets delayed sometimes by 5-10 minutes."

"Then what do you do?"

"I run the sterilisation cycle 5-10 minutes less. Say up to 20 minutes instead of 30. Actually 15 minutes at 121 degree is enough, you know.

"But the standard time is 30 minutes."

"So what?"

"So what means? Mr. Kanetkar always looks at the circular graph in the morning himself yaar. How come he never caught you?"

"You remember we used to do that frog leg experiment in the pharmacology lab?"

"Yeah, but what does that frog leg has to do over here?"

"Tell me, what we used to do when the frog leg doesn't respond properly?"

"Draw the line on the carbon bed paper with my hand."

"Exactly"

"What exactly? What do you mean?"

"Draw the line by hand for the remaining 10-15 minutes to show that you ran the cycle for 30 minutes. Simple yaar."

I was shocked at what my friend was doing, and also for trying to get me to do the same thing. This is something that NO PHARAMCIST SHOULD EVER DO, to catch the bus in time.

"Dinkar," I told him "even if I miss my bus all five days of the week I will never do this and since you are a very good friend of mine, I suggest that you don't do this either. This is like playing with people's lives, how can you not understand this?"

He had no answer. You must remember that we are supposed to be trained pharmacists, and "trained" means, one who has 1. Knowledge, 2. Skill and 3. A positive and constructive attitude towards the job.

Both of us had knowledge of sterilisation, both of us had the skill to operate the autoclaves but what about our attitude?

21

COLOURFUL AVIL EXPECTORANT

When I was working in the liquid oral department, I remember one incident, which explains the meaning of "managing by example."

Once I was manufacturing a batch of 'Avil expectorant,' a red coloured liquid oral preparation. The batch size was 1000 litres.

The red colour of the product was because of a combination of two colours.

I started manufacturing, the penultimate step was the addition of colour and final step was addition of flavour.

We used to make the colour solution in about 5 litres of purified water and then add it into the bulk. The actual colour of the product was bright red, i.e., when it gets diluted to 1000 litres, but in the 5 litres of water it was very dark. The operator dissolved the two colours in a small container containing about 5 litres of purified water, saw that the complete colour dissolves properly and then added the main bulk through a nylon cloth filter and stirrer kept for proper mixing and distribution. The flavours were also added, volume was made up to the required mark, and the batch was filtered and kept in the storage vessel.

The sample was sent to the Q.C. lab in an amber coloured bottle with a label. The batch was to be taken for filling the next day.

When I sent the sample it was about 2:30 P.M. At about 4:00 P.M. Mohan, our assistant Q.C. Manager called me to the lab. I did not know why I was summoned.

"Yes Mohan, did you call me?" I asked as I entered the Q.C. Lab.

"Yes Manohar, come here." Both of us entered Mr. Bhat's cabin, Mr. Bhat was our Q.C. Manager. He had two test tubes in the test tube stand. One of them had a red colour solution and in the other there was a dark amber coloured solution. (definitely not red)

"Yes sir?" I asked Mr. Bhat.

"Manohar, did you make this batch today?"

"Which batch sir?"

"Avil expectorant B. No XXX"

"Yes sir, I did." I replied.

"Have you checked the colour of the batch?"

"No sir."

"See this," he said as he pointed his finger towards the test tube containing the dark amber coloured solution.

"My god, how come that is the colour?"

"That is exactly what I am asking you!" Mr. Bhat's voice had changed, it had become quite rough. I got a little scared.

"I don't know sir, it shouldn't be this colour. I don't know what went wrong." I replied.

"Manohar and Mohan both of you go back to the department and take another sample and show me."

"Yes sir" we said as we left his room.

"Yaar Manohar, what is the problem? Kya lafda hai?" Mohan asked me on the way to the liquid department.

"I really don't know yaar, I am puzzled myself." I replied.

We collected another sample, came back to Mr. Bhat. The problem was true. The colour did not match the standardised bright red, but was same as that of the solution in the test tube–the dark amber coloured solution.

"Mohan hold the batch immediately, Manohar, give the batch papers and the raw materials labels to Mohan. Tomorrow we will see what is to be done."

"Yes sir," I said and left the room.

The entire next day was spent in investigating what went wrong. It was revealed that the stores dispensed a wrong colour. The production people never came to know that. During the dispensing, no production person was present there, only one dispensing pharmacist and one Q.C. chemist who used to check the dispensing.

On the third day Mr. Rajadhyaksha, the liquid department head, called me, the operators, the dispensing chemist who checked the dispensing, all from the liquid department.

When we entered, Dr. Ravi Rosha, production director, Dr. Hans Habischt, technical director and Mr. Bhat, the Q.C. manager were already in the department.

The whole scene was quite scary and tense. Dr. Habischt spoke in a very serious tone that, "This incident is a very serious quality failure and, the management has taken very strong steps in this regard, which you will know afterwards, but immediately we are discarding this batch, which costs the company Rs XX. This is a very unusual incident and you all should take a lesson from this. Remember the Hoechst stand on quality. Mr.. Bhat ask the operator to open the valve and drain the whole batch into the gutter, and don't leave the department till the whole batch has been drained. Is that clear?"

"Yes sir," Mr. Bhat replied.

Dr. Habischt left the department. We all were seeing the batch getting drained with our eyes wide open.

Lot of people were observing the whole high tension drama from behind the glass panes of the corridor.

Here by a single incident, Dr. Habischt showed us, what the management at Hoechst stands for and what quality meant for them.

22

DOUBLE DEFAULT IN VITA-HEXT

'Vita-Hext' was a very famous multivitamin liquid oral preparation, yellow coloured, which we used to manufacture.

We had our manufacturing vessel in a room exactly opposite to Mr. Shah's office, who was the manager of the liquid oral department.

At that time, there were two pharmacists working under Mr. Shah, Mr. Paranjyothi and I.

That day Mr. Paranjyothi was manufacturing Vita-Hext batch. The batch was in the final stage of manufacture i.e., making up the volume of the batch to 2000 litres, which was the batch size.

Our state excise inspector Mr. Joshi used to sit in the same room where we used to manufacture the batch, since our strong room was where we stored the alcohol.

Mr. Shah was sitting in his office, he called, "Mr. Paranjyothi, please come for a moment."

Paranjyothi looked into the vessel and saw that sufficient water was required to make up the volume to 2000 litres. He kept the purified water tap on and went to Mr. Shah's office.

Mr. Shah wanted to discuss some issue with him, they started discussing and Mr. Paranjyothi forgot that he left the water tap on.

"Paranjyothi, Paranjyothi," Mr. Joshi shouted at the top of his voice.

Mr. Shah and Paranjyothi got scared, and ran to the manufacturing room opposite his office.

What they saw, was that the entire department floor was fully flooded with Vita-Hext liquid over flowing from the manufacturing vessel.

"Paranjyothi, go and close the valve yaar." Mr. Shah shouted. Paranjyothi ran close to the valve. The whole floor was wet with the syrupy liquid. Pranjyothi could not keep his balance and slipped and fell. Mr. Joshi and Mr. Shah managed to help Paranjyothi. Meanwhile I slowly made my way to the valve and closed it. My shoes and the lower part of my trousers got drenched with the yellow coloured liquid of Vita-Hext.

I then gradually made my way to the vessel and closed the lid.

"Manohar, disconnect that main water pipe from the manufacturing vessel." Mr. Shah told me in an annoyed voice.

"Yes sir." I said.

Mr. Shah called a sweeper and asked him to get the whole department cleaned up. Paranjyothi went to change room to change his uniform. Mr.. Joshi closed the alcohol strong room. Mr. Shah while going to his office said, "Manohar, you and Paranjyothi please come to my room."

"Yes sir." I said.

I washed my shoes, tried to clean the lower part of my trousers and then went to Mr. Shah's office, Mr. Paranjyothi joined us in the meantime .

Mr. Shah was sitting in his chair, with both his palms covering his face. All three of us including Mr. Joshi were standing in front of him in his office.

Mr. Shah removed his palms from his face, rubbed his face a bit and then looked at us.

"Paranjyothi, what is this?"

"Sir actually….." I tried to explain.

"Manohar, let Paranjyothi talk to me."

"Yes sir." I said.

"Sir, actually I was making up the volume of the batch." Paranjyothi started to explain.

"So?"

"Sir, suddenly you called me."

"So?"

"I thought I will see you, go back and then make the volume up, since there was a lot of water required to make up the volume, so I kept the valve open."

"Then?"

"While I was talking to you I forgot and the tank overflowed sir. Sorry Sir." Paranjyothi was a little scared and a wee bit worried.

There was complete silence for a while. That was making us quite uneasy.

"How can we avoid such things? Who is going to explain all this to Dr. Rosha?

"Sir, it was my fault" Mr. Paranjyothi said with a low voice.

"Paran, that is not the issue. No one is going to hang for this, neither you nor me, but we cannot run the department like this."

"Sir, can I make a suggestion?" Mr. Joshi asked.

"Yes, Joshi saab, why not? I want a solution and I don't want something like this to happen again."

"Sir, I think, volume making is a critical operation, and the pharmacist should not leave this operation, even if anybody calls him. Or at least he should close the water connection and go, even if that means it'll take longer to make up the volume, it'll be worth it. What do you say Paran?"

"Yeah." Paranjyothi said.

"Joshi saab, I think your suggestion is correct, but I would like to add one more thing to this, to make it fool proof." Mr. Shah said.

"What is that sir?" I asked.

"Manohar and paranjyothi, both of you listen very carefully to what I have to say."

"Yes sir."

"We have a direct connection between the overhead purified water tank and the manufacturing vessel. Is it not?"

"Yes sir."

"This is very dangerous. I think we should disconnect that immediately and provide a flexible tube from the main tank to the manufacturing vessel and only when you require it you connect it, when not needed you remove it. So that we are safe. Because I remember sometime back, this valve had some problem. Even in the closed position it was leaking and the water kept dripping into product. Luckily there was not a major issue and we changed the valve and the problem was solved. But a risk of such leakage always hangs over us. What do you say Paran?"

"You are right sir."

"So what do we do now?"

"I will call Ceryl," Ceryl was our mechanic.

"Yes call him and get the direct water connection disconnected and provide a flexible hose okay?"

"Yes sir."

"Okay. Now close down the department. Tomorrow I will discuss with Mr. Mohan Kumar and will decide what to do with this batch okay?"

"Okay sir."

"Thank you Mr. Joshi, for your suggestion also. We will do both things." Mr. Shah thanked our state excise inspector. We then left Mr. Shah's room.

The next day we did the following things:

The batch was salvaged in the following manner.

(a)   The batch was divided into two equal parts.

(b)   Assayed for of all the ingredients used.

(c)   As a special care we dispensed the material exactly required for the batches based on the assay.

(d)   Reprocessed the batches.

(e)   A detailed deviation report was made by Mr. Shah and Mr. Mohan Kumar.

Secondly a decision was taken to disconnect the main purified water connection and use a flexible hose to make up the volume.

Next Mr. Shah gave very clear instructions to us that one should never leave one's place, when making up the volume, even if anyone calls you.

It was a nightmare, but we all learnt a valuable lesson from this.

We experienced another batch failure with Vita-Hext.

Vita-Hext contained vitamin B6 and B1 both. Since we used to make this product practically every day, the dispensing department used to weigh two batches at a time, to save time. While weighing, the dispensing pharmacist used to keep two containers side by side and weigh two units of each ingredient and put the bags one in each container.

One day I received two dispensed batches. I made one batch and sent the sample to Q.C.

Mr. Micheal was the analyst. He analysed the batch and called me to the lab.

"Yes Micheal?" I asked him.

"Yaar Manohar, this batch shows double B1"

"What?"

"Yes assay of B1 is double. 200% of what is expected. Kuch tho gadbad hai."

"How can it be yaar?"

"I don't know. Check from your side."

"Assay is correct na?"

"You are challenging my assay?"

"No, it's not like that, but you also check from your side, the dilutions and all you know."

"Manohar I have really checked everything, believe me, nothing is wrong from our side."

Meanwhile Mr. Mohan joined our discussion.

"Manohar, how many batches material you received today?" Mohan asked me.

"Two."

"So one batch, unused is still there with you?"

"Yeah."

"Micheal, come on, let's go and see if there is anything wrong with the materials." Mohan suggested.

All three of us came to our department. When we took out all the bags of vitamin from the container, we found to our surprise that this batch had two bags of vitamin B6 and no bags of vitamin B1.

We realised the problem. The dispensing pharmacist put two bags of vitamin B1 in one container and two bags of vitamin B6 in the other container. This mistake missed the scrutiny of the manufacturing pharmacist. (I was the manufacturing pharmacist)

Anyway, the batch was salvaged by making another batch with two hundred percent vitamin B6 and then mixing 50% of each, assaying and then filling.

23

TERRIBLE NOISE

I was making a batch of Avil syrup. The initial water was taken into the manufacturing vessel, the steam was started and stirrer was kept at a slow speed. I was waiting for the water to get heated up to 60-70 °C, before I could add the sugar.

The operator, asked me, "Sir please check the temperature. I think it must be above 60 °C." "Okay wait," I replied. I checked the temperature and asked him to start adding the sugar.

"Sir, why don't you come up on the platform. We will add the sugar by lifting the bag. We will add it slowly instead of using the scoop, it will be easier." He was trying to find a easier way out. I also agreed with him.

I got up there, we opened the bag, I supported it from the back side of the bag and he was at the open end of the bag, trying to control the flow of the sugar. In the good old days, "Vacuumax" like material transfer systems were not in use. It was all purely manual. The sugar was getting added slowly, suddenly the operator lost control of the open end of the bag and nearly one-fourth of the sugar in the bag got dropped in the vessel, and a terrible noise came from within the vessel. We did not understand what went wrong. Even if about 25 kg of sugar gets added it should not have produced such a noise. I left the bag and rushed to stop the stirrer. The noise also stopped.

Both of us were wondering what had caused the noise. To check once again I inched the stirrer and again the noise came. I stopped the stirrer and closed the steam connection. I also stopped the main electrical connection. We had a stainless steel rod about 6 feet long in our department. I asked the operator to bring that and asked him to slowly put it inside to try to see if something was lodged near the stirrer.

He put the rod in and tried to stir slowly by hand, we heard the noise again. There was definitely something inside. First of all, I thought that some part of the stirrer must have been broken or loosened and fallen inside. I asked the operator to call a mechanic immediately.

The operator ran to call the mechanic. After about ten minutes, the mechanic Ceryl came, "Potdar sab, what is the problem?" he asked. "Ceryl some unusual noise is coming from within when we start the stirrer."

He came up and inched the stirrer again and the same noise came.

By now the water had cooled and water vapours had subsided. Ceryl tried to peep inside from the manhole, but he could not see anything. The light inside the vessel also was not enough. He sent the operator to get the tiger torch from his room.

When the operator came back, he focussed the light from the tiger torch into the vessel. To his surprise he found an S.S. scoop at the bottom. "Potdar saab, there is a scoop inside." Ceryl said.

"What?"

"A scoop" Ceryl confirmed.

We managed to take the scoop out somehow. Ceryl inched the stirrer again. No noise came.

"Thank god." I said.

"But who dropped that scoop inside?" Ceryl asked.

"We don't know, we were adding the sugar from the bag, directly, without any scoop." I said.

Finally it was realised that the scoop was sealed inside the sugar bag itself. The sugar factory operator must have forgotten it inside and the bag must have been sealed with the scoop inside.

When we discussed this incident the following decisions were taken.

(a) No material will come to the production unit in supplier's sealed containers, even if it is sugar.

(b) No large quantity material will be added directly from the bag. Only small quantity material bags up to say five kg can be added directly from the dispensed bags.

Thank god! no major accident took place in this case, but we learnt a good lesson.

24

STORY OF CHLORAPHENICOL IN CATILAN CAPSULES

This is an incident that happened in the capsule department.

That time I was working in the capsule department. we had only two products namely; Catilan (Chloramphenicol capsules) and Hostacycline (Tetracycline HCl capsules).

We used to manufacture these products in campaign. The batch sizes were the same and small for both products.

That day Catilan campaign was to be manufactured. I had Rajayya Makili as an operator that day, who was a relatively new operator in the capsule section.

The procedure of manufacturing was that we used to sift all the batch ingredients in two containers, one after the other, and then fill them in a ball mill, add about 6 to 7 balls in the mill and close it and put it in the rotating cage.

We had two rooms in the capsule section, I used to sit in the filling room and the other room, we had sifting and blending activities.

"Rajayya, transfer the materials to the ball mill." I said.

"Yes sir," Rajayya replied.

Sometime lapsed, by then he should have transferred and filled the ball mill. I called him.

"Rajayya, what happened? You have still not loaded the ball mill?" I asked.

"Sir, the ball mill is full but there is still some material left over." Rajayya said.

"What?" I asked in surprise.

"Yes sir, the ball mill is full and there is still some material left be filled. What shall I do?"

"Are you sure?" I asked.

"Yes sir." Rajayya replied.

I had a doubt, probably Rajayya had mixed up some material of the second batch. But how could that happen? I myself had given him the batch material to be sifted and filled into the ball mill. I was worried. I went to the other room.

"Rajayya take two plastic bags." I asked him

He got two big bags.

"Weigh them."

"Okay sir," he weighed them, I recorded the weight.

"Rajayya let us fill all the sifted material into these two bags."

"Okay sir."

I helped him by holding the bags, while Rajayya put all the material into the two bags. We sealed the bags and weighed them one after the other and recorded the weight and checked how much is the net material.

To our surprise we found that the weight was correct, but then the volume was definitely substantially high. Now, I had a doubt, about the bulk density of the chloramphenicol. The material was supplied by Parke-Davis.

I asked Mr. Mohan about the bulk density of chloramphenicol, and explained to him the problem. He got worried.

He checked the bulk density, but said, "Manohar, we don't have a specification for bulk density in our raw material specification for chloramphenicol, so we don't check it."

Now we had a serious problem. I could have blended this batch in two lots but the desired quantity could not have gone into size one capsule. If we went in for a size zero capsule, we would be able to fill it with sufficient quantity of material but the entire packing would get affected. We had no choice but to get the material of the right bulk density.

The matter was taken to Mr. Bhat, our Q.C manager. He called the Parke-Davis people and complained about the change in the bulk density, which was substantially low. Parke-Davis manager said that he would check with his people and then call back.

Mr. Bhat received a call from Parke-Davis manager who said, "Our material meets the specification that you have given us. Since you did not have a specification for bulk density, it is not our responsibility. In fact the material that we have provided has a finer particle size and hence has a better therapeutic efficacy. However if you need a material of high bulk density, you give us the specification and we will meet it."

But we had a problem of what to do with the material that we already had with a low density. We still had quite a lot of material still lying in the stores. Mr. Bhat had a dialogue with the Parke-Davis people and the Parke-Davis people agreed to help us sort out the problem.

Finally a Parke-Davis fine chemicals chemist came to us. He suggested that we could compact the material using a role compactor, which luckily we had, and then mill it again. We did that and then got the material of the desired bulk density. We filled some of the capsules using this material and some excipients, tested the filled capsules specifications, found them to be okay and the problem got resolved.

We not only changed the specification of the chloramphenicol by adding bulk density specification in it, but also changed many more raw materials specifications, where this type of potential problem was expected.

25

PALLET IN THE RAIN

It was the beginning of rainy season, in the month of June.

Our capsule department was on the ground floor and behind our department there was an open space, from where there was a path to our central warehouse. The warehouse used to dispense the material batch wise and we used to bring the material and keep it in the open space on pallets, and the open space was open to the sky. Normally the material used to come between 3-4 P.M for the next day's production.

We had a summer trainee with us by name Govind Parayamalani, who had completed his B. Pharm and wanted to complete his two months training with us in May and June.

On that day the sky was cloudy and it could have rained at any time. The time was about four in the afternoon. It started to drizzle.

Dr. Ravi Rosha, our Production Director was coming from the warehouse towards our department, since there was a passage to go to his office from there.

He saw a young boy trying to use a pallet truck, probably to lift the material off the pallet and take it somewhere. But he did not know how to use the pallet truck properly. Dr. Rosha stopped there for a while and saw his efforts. The boy was trying all possible ways but still was unable to do it properly.

"Hey, what are you doing?" Dr. Rosha asked him.

He saw Dr. Rosha and got a little scared and replied, "Nothing sir, I was just trying to take this pallet to the capsule department."

"Why are you doing this yourself? Don't you have an operator in your department?"

"There is an operator sir, but at this moment he has gone for tea and it is drizzling, so the material will get wet if left here, so I was trying to take it inside."

"Who are you?" Dr. Rosha asked.

"College trainee sir. This week I am in the capsule department."

"Okay leave it, I will show you how to take the pallet out." Dr. Rosha lowered the pallet using the lever and pushed the fork inside the pallet, pressed the lifting device to lift the pallet and moved it.

"Thank you sir, I will do it now, I didn't know how to lower the fork. Now that I have seen you doing it, I will put the pallet inside." He said.

Parayamalani took the pallet inside. The material was saved from getting wet.

The next day morning Mr. Rajadhyaksha, our department head of capsules called me and said, "Manohar, what was the problem yesterday?"

"About what sir?" I asked.

"Did Parayamalani do something wrong with the materials?"

"No, I don't think so sir. Why, what is the problem?"

"I don't know Dr. Rosha met me in the morning and told me to come to his office at 10 A.M. along with Parayamalani."

"He is a good boy sir, very sincere in his work; I have been observing him for the last 4 days."

Mr. Rajadhyaksha and Govind went to Dr. Rosha's office at 10 sharp. I was quite worried about Govind.

At about 10:20 both Mr. Rajadhyaksha and Govind came back to the department. "What happened sir?" I asked, with uneasiness clearly visible on my face.

"Very serious," Rajadhyaksha said, with Govind still standing behind him.

"Tell me sir. What is it?" the eagerness was apparent in my voice.

"Govind has been appointed from 1st of July."

"What?" I saw a smile appearing on Govind's face and Rajadhyaksha started laughing.

"Really?" I asked.

"Yes sir." Govind told me.

"How come? What was that miracle?," I could not control myself. I shook hands with Govind.

"Manohar, Rosha saab had seen Govind trying to lift the pallet and take it into the department to save it from getting wet , as it was drizzling."

"So?"

"Rosha liked his concerned attitude towards the work and said, 'Raja, ask Bhende to recruit him as production supervisor."

"Oh my god! What an appreciation of work. Congratulations Govind."

"Thank you sir."

The story ends here. Govind was with us for quite some time, showing the same concerned attitude towards the work.

I do not think I need to say anything more about the incident.

26

BOSSE'S APRON

My boss Mr. Rajadhyaksha always used to wear a white half bush shirt. He would wear different coloured pants but never a change in the shirt colour or the style.

He used to come into the department change room, take out his white bush shirt and put on his white apron. Except the style, the colour looked the same as the shirt and it was impossible to recognise from a distance whether he was wearing a shirt or an apron.

In the department, our worker Chatar Singh used to look after laundry work of the department. This meant that he had to collect the soiled uniforms and aprons, put it into the laundry bag, send it to the central washing section of the laundry twice a week and collect it from the laundry collection section.

One day when the soiled clothes were to be given for washing, Chatar Singh was not there on duty, so I told another worker Gaikwad to collect the soiled clothes and send them to the laundry washing section. This was at about 3 o'clock in the afternoon. He did what I asked him.

Normally at about five in the evening we used to go to the change room to change our dress. Mr. Rajadhyaksha also used to be there.

We entered the change room. "Manohar, if you have done with your change, please put this apron there and get the bush shirt from the hanger," Mr. Rajadhyaksha said.

"Yes sir, give me that." He gave me the apron. I put it into the soiled clothes and started looking for his shirt. But I could not find it there.

"Sir, where did you put it?" I asked.

"At the usual place yaar, see on the hanger there."

"No sir, I don't see your shirt here."

"What?"

"Yes sir, I don't see it here." I repeated.

"Oh my god! Where did it go? How am I to go home now?" he said in a voice that was both annoyed and worried at the same time.

Meanwhile I saw Gaikwad coming into the change room.

"Gaikwad yaar where is Mr. Rajadhyaksha's shirt? Did you see it while giving the aprons for washing?" I asked.

"Sir's shirt? Where was it? I gave all the uniforms and aprons for washing from here."

"Oh my god!"

"Sir, probably your bush shirt was given for washing by Gaikwad, along with our laundry." I told Rajadhyaksha in a hushed tone.

"Oh my god, what nonsense! Gaikwad run to the laundry and get my shirt back." He shouted at him. Gaikwad ran to the laundry like an arrow released from the bow.

We were waiting in the change room for him to come back with the shirt.

Finally he came back empty handed.

"What happened? Where is my shirt?"

"Sir the laundry is already closed."

We did not know what to do. Finally I got an idea in my mind.

"Sir, I would have given you my shirt but that will be too loose for you. I feel today you can just wear your apron and tuck it inside your pant, nobody will know." I somehow put forth my idea.

He frowned at all of us standing there, but then he finally agreed.

"Okay give me that apron." He took it and put it on, and tucked it inside his pants. I helped him make the apron look somewhat like a shirt.

"Sir, I am really very sorry." Gaikwad said in a very uneasy voice. "I am very sorry, really very sorry." He repeated.

"Okay, okay. Take care in the future." He said to calm down Gaikwad.

"Manohar, it doesn't look odd? Does it?" he asked me.

"No sir, not at all." I said with complete confidence.

"Good! thank god for that. Good night."

He left the change room. Gaikwad saw that the boss had left through the half open door of the change room and then closed the door from inside.

"Gaikwad, you got saved today, but otherwise you had it" I said.

"Believe me sir, I really couldn't differentiate between sir's shirt and the aprons."

"I know"

"Now let us run, otherwise we will miss our bus." I shouted and we all ran to catch the bus.

27

CGMP AND CAP

It was the monthly production review meeting, which was normally attended by heads of departments and other senior managers. That day, Mr. Rajadhyaksha our head of the department was not present, so I had an opportunity to attend the meeting in his absence.

Various points were discussed in the meeting and the atmosphere in the meeting hall was getting a little tense due to some of the discussions.

Some points that were discussed were related to the implementation of cGMP. Meanwhile tea was served in the meeting. Dr. Rosha, who was chairing the meeting said, "let us have a small break, drink our tea and not discuss any business till then." After everyone had drunk the tea the meeting started again.

Mr. R.K. Shah was one of the heads of the department, opened the discussion after tea, "Sir, one of the things of cGMP is wearing a cap on the head, which is compulsory."

"Yes, I know that." Dr. Rosha said. "Why are you raising this point Shah?"

"Sir, I want some people to be exempted from this rule." Shah pleaded.

"What nonsense? Why? No, no, no, no! No one will be excluded from this Mr. Shah, no one. By the way whom do you have in mind? Dr. Habischt? He himself will not agree to your suggestion."

"No sir, not Dr. Habischt, I wanted Mr. Mithani and Dr. K.K. Maheshwari to be exempted sir."

"Why? What is so great about them? You know that the cap is a part of the uniform. It is to be worn to prevent hair falling into the product." Dr. Rosha put his point forward bluntly.

"That is what I am saying sir, for the both of them there is no chance of hair falling into the product. Don't you agree with me sir?" Shah answered with a mischievous smile on his face.

Dr. K.K. Maheshwari and Dr. Mithani both were completely bald. All the members of the meeting including Dr. Rosha savouned the naughtiness of the moment and the entire tension in the meeting vanished like a mist getting dispersed due to the bright rays of sunlight.

Dr. K.K. Maheshwari and Mithani joined the group, rubbing their bald heads with their palms.

28

TIKA ON FOREHEAD

It was Navarathri day, actually it was the day before Dassera.

The factory used to be closed on Dassera day hence every department used to have Dassera pooja on the earlier working day. In the factory canteen, on that day all the lady employees used to serve lunch and they used to be in their best dresses, sarees and accessories.

After the lunch the factory never used to work unofficially. All the people in the departments used to be busy with decorating their respective departments, with rangoli, flowers and whatever other way they could.

From about 3:30 P.M. all the seniors like Dr. Habischt, Dr. Rosha, Dr. K.K. Maheshwari etc. used to visit every department to meet the people.

At about 4:00 o'clock, they came to our department, the capsule section.

We welcomed them. We had a girl by name of Jaya Choudhari, who was a little short. She took the wet kumkum and put a large tika on the foreheads of Dr. Habischt, Dr. Rosha, and finally Dr. K.K. Maheshwari. She stretched the tika too far on his forehead and a little on his head.

"Hey Jaya, stop man, how long are you going to put the tikka on my head?" Dr. K.K. Maheshwari said. Dr. Rosha said in a jovial mood, though he was generally a very serious sort of person. "Krishna (Dr. Maheshwari's name), Potdar has probably told her to stop the tikka when she touches the hair on your head. But she is yet to touch them. So please don't blame her." Dr. Rosha said.

Everybody started laughing including Dr. Habischt and Dr. K.K. Maheshwari himself.

"I am sorry sir," Jaya said.

"It's all right Jaya, only intelligent people have this priviledge you know. Look at Dr. Rosha and Dr. Habischt, their head full of hair. You understand no, what I mean." Dr. K.K. Maheshwari said with a twinkle in his eyes and left Dr. Habischt and Dr. Rosha looking at each other.

29

NO JOB IS BIG OR SMALL, IT IS ONLY DIFFERENT

Time, eight thirty in the morning, I was in the factory canteen having my breakfast along with my colleagues.

"Sir, Sir, come quickly the entire department is full of water." Chatar Singh said requesting me to come to the department immediately.

"How come? What happened? Where did the water come from?" I raised many questions, while taking my last sip of tea.

"Shyam, I am going" I said to my colleague Shyam Khante who was from the antibiotics department, who always used to give me company for breakfast.

"Should I come with you?" Shyam asked.

"No, no, don't worry, I will manage. Come, Chatar Singh." I said and both of us rushed to the department.

I saw the entire floor was wet with water. Being the capsule department this was very risky.

I picked up the intercom and tried to call the maintenance department. Nobody picked up.

I sent Chatar Singh to the workshop to find somebody and also tried to contact housekeeping staff.

Being tea time, I literally could not get anyone on line. I realised that the water was coming from the drain of the liquid department, which was exactly on top of the capsule department.

I called Mr. Shah and told him, he stopped washing of the liquid vessels so the water would not go down to the capsule department. The flow of water stopped but whatever water was already in the department needed to be removed fast. I was trying to contact housekeeping staff frantically, but without any success.

At this juncture suddenly Dr. Rosha entered the department. He found the entire floor of the department fully wet. He looked at the hygrometer, the humidity was very high and then he looked at me and said, "Hey, what is happening? From where has all this water come?"

I told him the story.

"Then what are you doing? Have you seen the humidity in the department?"

"Yes sir."

"Then what are you doing?" He asked again.

"I am trying to contact the housekeeping staff sir, but nobody is responding." I said giving my excuse.

"Do you have a floor scrapper?"

"Yes sir."

"Where is it?"

I showed him the rubber floor scrapper.

He took that in his hand and ordered, "Open that middle door." I did that.

He started to clear the water by using the housekeeping's rubber scrapper.

"Sir, why are you doing this? The housekeeping will be here and they will do it sir." I said while trying to take the scrapper from his hand.

"Are you going to wait till the sweeper comes or are you going to do it?" he asked.

I did not know what to say. I managed to say, "No sir, I will do it myself."

Meanwhile Chatar Singh also managed to get another scrapper and started removing the water. "That is good. Manohar, never wait in situations of emergency to do a job. Don't ever think that a job is inferior or something. Remember no job is small or big, they are only different and you should be able and willing to do it if required."

"Yes sir." I said.

The flood in the capsule department gave me a very very important lesson, that "No job is small or big, it is only different." That was when I realised if Dr. Rosha can do this job then why can't I?

30

THE HOSTACYCLINE MYSTERY

In our capsule department there were only three products at that time i.e., Hostacycline, Catilan and Jonit. Out of the three Jonit capsules were made in a separate section while Hostacycline (Tetracycline) and Catilan (Chloramphenicol) were manufactured in one section on a campaign basis i.e., we used to finish a month's production of Hostacycline, say about 50-60 batches, clean the entire department, including the equipment and then start the Catilan manufacture, and make about 30-40 batches of the same. This was the regular practice.

Earlier I was looking after this work. Later Mr. Athawale, another pharmacist started looking after this section. In that particular month he was first manufacturing the Hostacycline batches.

We were manufacturing only one product at a time and that too for a long time, since batches used to be a campaign. The cleaning of the filling machine was not a very thorough process. Once a week we used to have a thorough cleaning by dismantling the filling machine and all the other equipment. Batch to batch contamination/ mix-up was really not given due consideration. (Don't ask me about the cGMP's strict adherence etc.)

We had a good powerful, 3-head 'Delstar' vacuum cleaner attached to the GKF-700 capsule filling machine which used to suck the powder from around the filling turret and other sides of the machine.

We used to transfer the filled capsules to the packaging department. The batch quantity used to be seventy thousand capsules and the transfer was by weight of the seventy thousand capsules. We used to make the blend of each batch and put it into a plastic bag in an aluminium container. The empty capsules we used to get in lump sum for a part or the full campaign.

The blends were made ready sufficiently in advance. Filling used to go on continuously and the filled batches used to be sent to intermediate store as and when they were ready.

The campaign was going on smoothly and had practically come to an end. Mr. Athawale was taking an account of the whole campaign. He realised that all the blended batches were over but one batch of empty capsules was still remaining and also one batch of filled capsules was not transferred to the intermediate store. This simply meant that one batch of Hostacycline blend was missing. He searched the department but could not find it. He was a relatively new pharmacist and he checked the B.P.C.R's. It was clearly indicated that the batch was blended by him. He literally got scared. First he came to me, we both checked the things again but the situation was same, both of us got a little worried. We went to Mr. Rajadhyaksha and narrated him the story.

We thought he would also get worried and maybe he would reprimand us. But he was quite cool. "Sir what do we do? Where could the material have gone?" I asked.

"Athawale, tell me when did you clean the Delstar vacuum cleaner last?" was his cool question to Athawale.

"No sir, I have not cleaned the Delstar since the campaign started. I thought I would clean it at the end." Athawale answered.

"That means you have not cleaned the Delstar for the past fifteen days?" I asked.

"No Sir."

Rajadhyaksha looked at me and I realised where the blend was, "Sir, I know where the batch is."

"Athawale go down, your entire batch is in the Delstar," Rajadhyaksha shouted.

Both of us went down and asked the operator to open the Delstar vacuum cleaner and we found about 35 kg of Hostacycline was lying in that big three-headed Delstar vacuum cleaner.

You know what happened, the delstar is a powerful vacuum cleaner. Athawale never cleaned it during the entire campaign. Ideally it should be cleaned after every batch, if not at least after only a few batches. The recovery of all the 40-50 batches was lying in the Delstar. (What about cGMP?)

Thereafter we decided to clean the Delstar after each batch irrespective of whether the campaign was completed or not.

The days were passing like this in Hoechst. We were enjoying our job, lunch, company of people and everything. I never realised where nearly eight years had passed.

I left Hoechst to join Boehringer Knoll as Production Manager and a new career started for me as a Manager. But the best time in my entire career was the eight years I spent at Hoechst, which I loved, as I used to interact with my workers directly. Some of the close workers names I still remember, like Chatar Singh, Gaikwad, Tatoba, Rajayya Makili, Blaze Colaso, Pushpkadam, Laxmi, Kamal, Mithilda Rodrigues and Liz (Elizabeth), and also my collegues and seniors like Dr. Habischt, Dr. Rosha, Dr. K.K. Maheshwari, Mr. Bhat, Mr. Rajadhyaksha, Lata, Micheal, Athawale, Khante, and many more.

It was a really memorable span of time.

31

NOVALGIN-BARALGAN COMPRESSION

Novalgin and Baralgan were two very popular tablet products in Hoechst.

Novalgin had analgin in it and Baralgan had two other active substances in it, one was a Ketone and the other was an amide. (The chemical names were very complicated, we all used to call them Baralgan-amide and Baralgan-ketone.)

The tablet department used to work in two shifts; we had a shift register in which we normally used to write instructions, for the next shift supervisor if any. The batch sizes of the Novalgin and Baralgan were very large, and the compression of one batch used to go in two shifts and sometimes maybe even more than that. The tablet weights of Novalgin and Baralgan were very close. The shape and size was the same, one face was also the same and only the other was different.

When we used to go from a batch of Novalgin to Baralgan, we used to change only one set of punches which were different, because dies and one set of punches was common.

One day the production of batches of Novalgin was completed at about ten in the morning. The next batch was of Baralgan. The punches of Novalgin used to be removed and replaced with the punches of Baralgan. The machine was cleaned and kept ready for changing the punches. But suddenly the boss allotted the operator some other job and asked him to change the punches later. He said, "The Baralgan batch has to be taken in the afternoon, and you have sufficient time in between, when you can do this."

The operator left the job half way. I was busy with transferring the compressed batch of Novalgin to the intermediate store. I did the transfer and left for lunch. After coming from lunch, I confirmed that the granules of the Baralgan batch are received. I checked the weight, it was alright.

I looked at the watch, it was two thirty. I thought of writing my instructions to the second shift supervisor. I wrote that the Novalgin batch is completed, the Baralgan granules are checked and kept in the department and you can start the Baralgan compression when you come.

The second shift supervisor read instructions and started compressing the batch of Baralgan (IPQC was really not very strict back in the 70's, production supervisors used to start the production many a times without waiting for clearance from IPQC.)

After compressing about a few thousand tablets, suddenly the operator realised that the punches of Novalgin here have not been changed and the Baralgan batch was being compressed as Novalgin tablets.

He stopped the machine and informed the supervisor. He checked the register. He found no instructions about changing the punches. He thought the Baralgan punches have already been put. The whole issue came to light, only after the operator realised the mistake.

The production was stopped, compressed tablets collected, quarantined them, Novalgin punches were removed and finally the Baralgan punches were put. The tablets that were already punched were crushed, analysed and cleared by Q.C lab and the batch was restarted the next day.

Lesson from this was very clear;

- Never start a production batch without I.P.Q.C clearance
- "Write and read" the shift instructions very clearly.
- Never take anything for granted.

32

GO-SLOW

I joined Boehringer Knoll in 1980 as a Production Manager. My responsibility was to look after their centralised packing department.

Nineteen seventy three to nineteen eighty I was working with Hoechst India Ltd. in formulation manufacturing but did not have any experience of packaging. This was my first exposure in the pharma packaging as Manager.

The main difference between manufacturing and packaging from the managerial point of view is the number of people you handle. So far I had not handled a very big crowd of people any time since in manufacturing, in any section you generally do not have more number of people. I had handled only small groups of ten to twenty people at the most. But as a packaging Manager in the centralised packaging department I had more than hundred workers under my charge and two officers and two team leaders as well. Team leaders were very senior capable workmen. One of them was Mr. Shetty and another was Mr. Ambekar. The officers were Mr. Vasant Kabad, a relatively senior officer and the other officer was Mr. Amar Bhagt, a smart, young, dynamic, but very sober and decent person.

I joined this company in May 1980, at a time when some industrial relations issues were going on. The labour union was very strong. The union general secretary was Mr. Damu Shelake and his associate was Mr. Bhosale. Bhosale was working with my section in liquid packaging department. Even though he was a worker, he was a graduate in sociology and that time pursing law.

There was a major issue going on related to low productivity and bonus payments for the workmen.

To tackle the low productivity issue the company had hired Bombay Productivity Council for carrying out work study in the company and they had started with packaging department. There was always a difference of opinion on the productivity issues, and the workers representatives and the management representatives were always opposed to each other. The working environment was very tense. The production was not coming upto the mark. The management representatives were also tense. Incidentally I was one of the management representatives on the team.

It was a totally new experience for me. Luckily Mr. Shetty and Mr. Ambekar, though working on behalf of the workers group, were pro-management. They always tried to boost production but they also had pressure from the workers to reduce production.

The entire situation in the factory was not congenial and every day the tension kept mounting.

Finally the workers resorted to the technique of "Go-slow" (This refers to the typical tactic of the workers union to reduce production in such a way that it will not be possible for the managers to prove that the reduced production is because of the workers).

Alternately management decided to declare "Lock-out" i.e., stoppage of work and closing the factory till the labour management issues are solved amicably. It required, at that time, as per law, a notice of 15 days, which was also served by the management. The labour union went to the labour court in Thane. The case was heard in the labour court by a judge called Mrs Gaitonde.

Everyone in the factory, including the workmen were now in a tense and gloomy mood.

One day I called Mr. Damu Shelake and Bhosale to my cabin. Damu refused, but Bhosale being a worker of my department came. I also called Shetty and Ambekar, and started the following dialogue,

"Mr. Bhosale, you know that the management had declared a "lock-out" and after fifteen days the company will be closed. The workers and the management staff; both will suffer."

"I know sir."

"From tomorrow, we have the hearing in the labour court in front of Mrs Gaitonde."

"Yes sir."

"I really don't know what will happen there, but all of us will end up suffering. It is going to be a very bad situation for all of us." I continued.

"What can we do sir? Management is not agreeing to our demands." Bhosale said.

"Damu is not ready to talk to the management. Really speaking Damu has to speak to the management. Management is willing to resume dialogue."

"But sir Damu is general secretary of the union."

"I know, but you are the only person who can convince Damu to engage in a dialogue with the management." I suggested to Bhosale.

"I will talk to him, but I have my own doubts, I don't think he will agree."

"Why don't you try at least."

"I will" Bhosale promised and left the room.

The labour union refused to talk to the management and the case started in labour court. The case was to be heard every day for about one week; that is what Mrs Gaitonde told both the parties.

I was to attend the labour court as management representative along with our company advocate.

On the first day, I was going to court; the company advocate was to come there directly. I was sitting in the company car. I crossed the gate and came out onto the road, the car turned to the right, I found Mr. Bhosale and two more union representatives standing near the bus stop in front of our factory. I asked the driver to stop the car.

"Hey Bhosale, why are you waiting here?" I asked.

"To go to the court sir."

"How are you going?"

"By bus sir."

"Why don't you join me? I am also going there only."

He hesitated for a while and then said,

"No sir, you please carry on by car, we will come by bus." Bhosale said.

"Why? Come, come." I forced them to come into the car. We all travelled in the company car to the court. When we reached the court premises and were getting out of the car, Mrs Gaitonde's car also entered the court premises.

She saw Bhosale and me getting down from the same car, we greeted her and went inside. There was a surprised smile on her face.

The case continued for 3-4 days, arguments and counter arguments were going on. We used to go to court by the same car and come back to the company after the hearing, also by the same car. Mrs Gaitonde observed that we were coming and going by the same car.

On the fourth day she called me to her chamber and told that tomorrow I want Dr. Amonkar to come to the court. Dr. Amonkar was our factory head.

I communicated the message to him. He came to the court at sharp ten in the morning the next day.

Dr. Amonkar and I entered the Mrs Gaitonde's chamber. We greeted each other

"Dr. Amonkar, I would like to tell you an observation of mine."

"What is that ma'am?"

"My many years of experience says that your management and workers really have no issues. You can resolve what little differences you have, sitting here in my chamber.

"I will be very happy ma'am to solve it in an amicable manner. I too am not interested in this court business. If you can help us, I am prepared to settle it in your presence."

"That is wonderful. Can you call in the union representatives?"

"Yes ma'am." I said and went to call Damu and Bhosale. All three of us entered her chamber.

"Sit down, sit down all of you." Mrs Gaitonde said.

Next thirty minutes the discussion went on very amicably between Dr. Amonkar and Mrs Gaitonde and Mr. Damu Shelake.

After the meeting Dr. Amonkar asked her, "Ma'am tell me how did you conclude that there is actually no issue?"

"My one single observation made me conclude that."

"What was that?" Dr. Amonkar asked.

"Your production Manager and your union representatives coming to court in the same car, and I did not see any rivalry on their faces."

"Oh I see, that is true ma'am." Dr. Amonkar said, finally thanked her and left.

The issue of the go-slow and lock-out both were resolved, and we came out from Mrs Gaitonde's chamber with a big smile on our faces.

From this one experience I learned that many of the labour management issues can be resolved by real understanding of each other. Ultimately love-affection and business can go together. Throughout my remaining career as a manager this attitude always helped me.

33

ENTHUSIAM VS PRACTICALITY

In the 70's promotions in the industry used to be very slow. It used to take ten to twelve years to become a manager. When I became a manager seven years after my M. Pharm I was feeling really good and proud too. After M. Pharm I had completed D.B.M. from Mumbai. In my new job as manager I was really bubbling with enthusiasm, because I found that it was a really good opportunity to showcase my talent both as a pharmacist and manager both.

I found the materials management aspects related to issues of packaging materials from the warehouse and receiving by packaging department and then returning the packaging materials from the packaging department to warehouse had lot of problems and there was a lot of confusion in these transfers. This was resulting in confusion in the accounting of the materials too. These accounting issues were reflecting as inefficiency and un-systematic working of packaging department. Since now I was looking after this department as manager, I was very upset about the way things were being run.

I decided to streamline these operations. I prepared a lengthy document on A4 size papers for reconciliation of all the packaging materials of each batch, including receipts, consumption, rejection, and returns of these materials. The warehouse manager, the packaging materials dispensing executive, packaging department and I were supposed to fill various details in that. I thought that it will definitely streamline the packaging materials management system. I was very happy. I got cyclostyled about fifty such forms for immediate implementation and went to Mr. V.P. Samant, my boss, who was the works manager to show him the new system that I had devised.

"Good morning sir," I greeted Mr. Samant.

"Good morning, good morning, come, come." He welcomed me.

"Thank you sir."

"Yes? Anything special?"

"Sir as I told you last week there are some issues related to the packaging materials management system and our department is blamed for that."

"Yes I know you told me that."

"Sir I have made a new format, this will track the whole movement of the materials right from the stores to us and back again."

"Wonderful. So?"

"I want to implement this system sir."

"Good, show me that."

I enthusiastically showed him the forms that I had made.

"Yes they are good. Very detailed."

"Yes sir, I have not left out anything. This format is for every batch sir."

"Every batch?" he asked with a big question mark on his face.

"Yes sir, every batch." I replied again very enthusiastically.

"Who is going to fill this?"

"All the concerned people sir."

"Hmm! have you discussed it with them?"

"No sir."

He looked at me with his eyebrows raised.

"How much time will it take?"

"I don't know sir, I have not yet checked, but whatever time it takes, it is necessary, isn't it, sir?" I looked at him for his approval.

"Have you ever tried this at least on a trial basis?"

"No sir."

He smiled and I found it hard to understand the meaning of his smile.

"What happened sir?" I asked very innocently.

"Okay, do one thing, run the system on a trial basis for the next ten days and then come to me," he said.

"Okay sir."

"Good, proceed." I left his room and went back to the department.

Next ten days I tried my best to implement "my" system but failed miserably.

One day Mr. Samant called me and asked, "Any progress Manohar?"

"No sir."

"Why? What happened?"

"People here are very resistant sir, they just don't want to implement "my" system." I explained.

He looked me straight in the eyes and said, "Sit down"

I sat down in front of him.

"Do you know why they resist Manohar?"

"No, not really." I confessed.

"Because you say it is "your" system, Make it "their" system and then you will find "they" will accept it." I could not quite understand the meaning of Mr. Samant's statement.

"What does that mean sir?"

"Simple, now carefully listen to what I say?" I sat back and listened to him attentively.

"Yes Sir."

"See, the first thing you have to keep in mind is that, the system should look like "their system" and not "your system". You should be able to sell your idea to all those people who are involved and who are going to be affected by your system." He took a pause and continued.

"Go to them, (don't call them) discuss with them by explaining, what is the present issue, what we should do to improve the situation, how it will be beneficial for "them", the company and finally to "all". Never utter anything about how it is going to benefit you, never."

"Suggest your system, do not force it. Take their suggestions on the system. There may be some good suggestions coming from them. Some changes, some alterations, additions that may have to be made. Do not reject any idea or suggestion point blank, think them over. Create an environment where they will feel you are their man, who wants to do something for their benefit, to their advantage to make their job easier. Then trial run the discussed, modified and agreed upon system. After the trial run discuss the results, the positives and the negatives of the system with them very frankly. They will be happy. Then take their comments and try to implement "their" system and it will get implemented."

"Never say "my", similarly "give" credit to all of them, saying "their" system is really working. In all probability they will tell you, "no sir it is actually your system and it is working very well.""

"If you give credit where credit is due, then credit will automatically come back to you. Do you understand?"

"Yes sir. Thank you for all your guidance. This is something that I never read in books."

He smiled at me warmly and I left his room with my newly regained enthusiasm.

34

LEAVE APPLICATION

When I joined Boehringer Knoll as a Manager of the packaging department, I had two officers working with me, one was Mr. Vasant Kabad, a relatively senior officer, in fact he was older than me, and the other officer was Mr. Amar Bhagat who was a young officer. Both of them were BSc graduates and were working in that position for a long time.

I found no problem with Mr. Amar Bhagat but Mr. Vasant did not like the fact that I joined that department, because he felt like his prospects were getting sealed because of me. This was why he was keeping a sort of distance from me, and trying to undermine me as his superior. Earlier he was reporting to my boss Mr. Samant and now he was asked to report to me, so he was finding it humiliating and uncomforting.

In the month of May 1981, he wanted to go on privilege leave for about three weeks. He was supposed to send that application to me for approval, but he did not want to do that because sending me that application would mean that he was accepting me as his boss, which he did not want to do. So he sent his leave application directly to Mr. Samant for approval. By this he wanted to show that he does not accept me as his boss.

Since two days had passed and he still had not got his application back from Mr. Samant, he was starting to get a little uneasy. On the third day he was called by Mr. Samant to his room and Mr. Samant gave his application back to him unsigned, and said to him, "You need not send that to me anymore, you have to get it approved by Mr. Potdar."

Mr. Vasant had no choice but to come to me with his application for approval.

Mr. Samant had discussed this situation with me beforehand. Mr. Samant said, "Mr. Potdar, Vasant is such a good officer, but he finds your appointment as a hurdle to his progress, and that is quite a normal behaviour for any human being. He will take some time to come back to normal and accept you as his superior, but you don't worry. I have asked him to send his application to you. He will come to you, discuss with him his leave plan, talk to him in general and then approve his application."

I understood Mr. Samant's advice and when Vasant came to me with his leave application, I followed Mr. Samant's advice and then approved his leave application.

Over a period of time he also understood the situation and gradually we began to work together harmoniously as a team.

What I liked here was the way Mr. Samant handled the situation, without hurting the ego of either one of us, but at the same time maintaining the line of command intact. We do face such situations in corporate life and it must be resolved amicably, just like in this case.

35

HUNGER STRIKE

My days with Boehringer Knoll were during the most turbulent days of the company. There used to some problem or other due to labour unrest.

During one of these days, I was in my room, which was attached to the central packaging hall. My charge hand Mr. Ambekar came to me looking a little worried.

"Sir the union has decided to boycott the lunch from the canteen today." Ambekar said.

"Boycott? What does that imply?"

"Union General Secretary has told all the workmen, not to go to the canteen for lunch today."

"Why?"

"I really don't know but this must be one of their ways to press their demands, what else?"

"Ambekar can you call Bhosale?"

"Yes sir." Ambekar went to call Mr. Bhosale who was on the ground floor. It was about twelve thirty in the afternoon.

I called the canteen Manager to find out if he knew about the situation and was prepared for it and had anybody come for lunch.

He replied, "Sir the food is already prepared, no workmen came to lunch but some supervisory staff are in there having their lunch right now."

"Okay" I said.

That means food for more than 200 persons was ready and if no workers were going to take lunch then all of it would go waste. I was thinking about how to avoid this wastage.

"May I come in sir?" Bhosale asked from outside.

"Yes, come in Bhosale, sit down."

"Thank you sir." Bhosale sat down in the chair in front of me.

I did not say anything. I was sitting very quietly and playing with a paper weight on my table. I looked at him and he started to get a little uncomfortable.

"You called me sir?"

"Bhosale what is the problem suddenly?"

"About what sir?"

"As if you don't know. Tell me why have you people boycotted lunch?"

He did not give me any answer but had a very uneasy look on his face.

"Food for over two hundred people has been prepared and you people have advised your workmen not have food. Do you know what the wastage will be? And how will people work without lunch till they reach home, at about six thirty - seven in the evening? What are you people doing Bhosale? I don't understand. Is this the way a responsible union person like you should behave? Tell me what do you expect to do with the food of those two hundred people? Find a reasonable way to press your demands to the management. I know at least that you are not the type of person to use such tactics. Am I right or not? Tell me."

"All this is not in my hands sir. Damu is adamant; I may not be able to convince him at all. Would you like to talk to him sir?" Bhosale asked me.

"No. I am not going to talk to him. He will not listen. He is not at all a reasonable person. Okay, you may go Mr. Bhosale, but see that there is no untoward incidents. My officers may be taking their lunch there."

"Don't worry sir. Nothing untoward will happen. I am there in the canteen."

"Thanks."

"Okay sir." Bhosale said and left my room.

Time passed. It was about two thirty. Normally Mr. Sawant, Mr. Vyas, our manufacturing manager, and I used to go to lunch normally at about one thirty - two. But today none of us went for lunch."

At about two forty or so, I heard a knock on my door.

"Come in." I said.

Damu and Bhosale entered my room. I looked at Damu with my eyebrows raised. After a pause I said, "Sit down Damu, sit down, Bhosale please sit down."

"It is okay sir." Damu and Bhosale remained standing in front of my desk.

"Yes? What can I do for you?"

"Sir, you did not come to lunch today, neither did Mr. Vyas nor Mr. Sawant. The food is getting cold."

I looked at Damu, "Did you have your lunch?" I asked.

"We are not going to have it today sir."

"So are we."

"What is your problem sir? Why can't you people have your lunch?" Damu asked.

"Our boys have not taken food, then how do you expect us to have it? Tell me?"

"Our problem is different sir. You please have your lunch. I have asked the canteen manager to send you food here."

"Damu, please stop him. We are not going to have lunch until you people have it. Whatever is the problem we can always discuss and resolve it. We are always doing that." I said.

"Damu, sir is right, I think…." Damu stopped Bhosale midway and said, "Bhosale, Okay all of us will go to the canteen after fifteen minutes. I will talk to the canteen manger and arrange for lunch." Damu said.

Bhosale ran to tell the workmen. "Sir you always say that I am adamant, but you are equally adamant. Okay sir, I am sending your lunch here."

"No Damu wait."

"What is the problem now?"

"Don't worry. There is no problem. We will join you in the canteen for lunch. Let me tell Mr. Samant and Vyas. I will be waiting for you to come for lunch in the canteen."

"Okay" Damu replied and left the room.

My experience through more than thirty five years of industrial career was that people are generally good. The only thing they need is a bit of understanding.

36

CASE OF CALCILUVIN

It was my day one in Boehringer Knoll. Mr. Samant, our works manager and I were having tea in his room. It was about eleven thirty or so.

Mr. Samant's intercom rang.

He answered, "Yes Mr. Samant."

"Sir, drug inspector Mr. M. P Pore is coming to see you in your office. I have sent Mr. Jagdish with him." Our security officers voice at the other end.

"Okay, Okay I am coming," said Mr. Samant.

He then said to me, "Mr. Potdar, drug inspector Mr. Pore is coming. I don't know what he is like, let us receive him."

"Who is coming?"

"Mr. M. P Pore."

"Probably I know him. I think he is from my college."

"Good, if that is so then I can leave him to you."

"No problem sir," I said.

Jagdish, our security person entered the room with Mr. Pore.

"Good morning Mr. Samant, I am Mr. M.P Pore, drug inspector." Mr. Pore introduced himself.

"Welcome sir, welcome. Please take your seat." Mr. Sawant welcomed him.

"Hi Manohar. What are you doing here?" Pore asked me.

"Hi, I work for Boehringer Knoll. In fact today is my first day in this company."

"Oh that is good."

"What would you like to have sir? Tea? Coffee? Cold drink?" Mr. Samant asked.

"Anything will do." Mr. Pore answered while sitting down on the chair.

I went out and asked Ganesh to get some tea and entered the room again.

"Mr. Samant, I have received a market complaint about your product Calciluvin syrup from Jaipur." Pore went straight to the subject.

"Complaint? What complaint?" Samant's face showed some worry. His forehead showed some wrinkles.

"Ants."

"Ants?"

"Yes. There were ants in the bottle with the Calciluvin inside. The bottle is perfectly sealed."

"My god! How can that be?"

"I too am not convinced. Initially I thought it must be a fabricated case, but Mr. Samant the bottle seems to be genuine. No pilferage is seen." Pore put the bottle in front of Mr. Samant.

I looked at the bottle with curiosity. Yes, there were a few, maybe five or six dead ants floating inside the calciluvin syrup. I gave the bottle to Mr. Samant. He too observed it closely.

"Hmm yes there are," Samant responded.

He looked very carefully to the skirting of the ROPP cap and its bridges, they looked genuine.

"Yes, there is a problem Mr. Pore, the bottle really looks genuine." Mr. Samant continued.

"That's what I also think. The problem is really serious. I don't know how it happened." Pore remarked.

"We have to go into it in detail." Mr. Samant assured

"Mr. Samant I would like to see your bottle washing and liquid processing area."

"Oh by all means."

"I will call Mr. Vyas, our manufacturing manager." Mr. Samant picked up his intercom.

While we were wondering how this could have happened, Mr. Vyas entered the room. Mr. Vyas a fairly senior person in his late forties, thin, tall, with a full white apron and a cap with typical elderly spectacles.

"Mr. Vyas meet Mr. Pore, drug inspector." Samant introduced Mr. Pore to Mr. Vyas.

"Good morning sir." Mr. Vyas greeted.

"Good morning."

"Mr. Vyas, Mr. Pore has a gift for all of us." Samant said in a lighter mood to ease the tension that was slowly mounting in the room. Everyone laughed. The tension really vanished but the problem still remained.

Mr. Samant explained the issue to Mr. Vyas and asked him to show Mr. Pore whatever he asks for. "Mr. Pore, Mr. Vyas will take you to the department. I will be waiting for you here. Once you finish, we will meet again. Is that okay?"

"Sure." Mr. Pore replied.

"Potdar why don't you join us?" Mr. Pore asked me.

I looked at Mr. Samat and Mr. Vyas alternately.

"Of course why not? Mr. Potdar please join them."

And then the three of us left the room.

For the next hour or so we moved through the bottle receiving, bottle washing, bottle storage for washing, liquid manufacturing, liquid filling, packing and all the other relevant areas. Mr. Pore was making some notes in his visits diary.

We came back to Mr. Samant's room after an hour.

"Any clue Mr. Pore?" Mr. Samant asked.

"Probably, I think I know where the problem lies."

"Really?"

"Yes."

"Why don't you share your observations and findings." Samant requested Mr. Pore.

We all became very attentive as Mr. Pore began to explain to us his findings.

"You have a bottle washing machine down there, where it washes bottles using purified water but you don't wash the bottles by brushing. I understand for the fresh bottles it may not be required."

"However you recover some of the bottles as filled rejection. These bottles are rewashed and used again for bottle filling operation, which is also perfectly acceptable. I saw a tray of bottles which were recovered from the filling section after emptying the syrup. The bottles were lying in the washing section for the last two days, because the last two days were your weekly off."

"Your operator told me that these bottles will be washed today in the afternoon, on the same machine which is being used for the fresh bottles."

"I observed some bottles in the recovered bottles tray and I found some traces of syrup stuck inside on the surface of the bottles some dried up syrup. We put some of the bottles from the recovered bottle tray into the washing cycle for the fresh bottles and then checked to see whether they got washed thoroughly. We kept these bottles upside down to drain the water and then observed them. We still found some traces of dried up syrup inside, that means that the bottles were not getting thoroughly washed."

"To our surprise we found at least two bottles with some dead ants inside stuck to the surface along with the dried up syrup. Here are those bottles. You can have a look at them Mr. Samant." Mr. Pore said and then passed the bottles having the dead ants inside them over to him.

"Yes, you are right Mr. Pore". It is a problem. We must find a solution for it." Mr. Samant said.

"I have one or two suggestions to make." Mr. Pore said.

"Yes of course, your suggestions are always welcome." Mr. Samant told Mr. Pore with full genuine respect for his suggestions.

"Mr. Samant, you have a brush washing machine down there. You can use that for washing the recovered bottles. Other fresh bottles you can continue to wash using your present machine. The second thing is, please do not keep the recovered bottles for so long without washing, because the dried syrup is difficult to wash out. Make it a practise to clean these recovered bottles every day. In case of the weekends you may keep these bottles dipped in water, if you are not able to do the washing the same day. This will avoid scaling up of the bottles by dried syrup inside the bottle."

And most important is that your pest control should be much better than what it is presently. There cannot be even a single ant or any other pest for that matter in the processing, washing or storage area. I am really not at all happy about this situation."

Mr. Pore put his observation and suggestions very bluntly and straight to us.

"I appreciate your observations and remarks Mr. Pore. They are very useful to us and I can assure you that your suggestions will be immediately acted upon, I am advising your friend Mr. Potdar to implement these and you will be kept posted about it." Mr. Samant assured Mr. Pore.

"Okay, that is good. However I have to make my report on this investigation and submit to my boss, a copy of the same will be sent to you also. Meanwhile I need your signatures on my today's observations." Mr. Pore talked like a typical government officer on duty.

"Yes of course, my only request to you Mr. Pore is that keep our genuine acceptance and assurance given to you for implementing your suggestions, while making the final report. We always believe in F.D.A officer's educative approach." Mr. Samant spoke like a trained factory Manager.

"I know, and now that Mr. Potdar is there with you, I believe that your assurance is genuine and I expect no more complaints from your plant. I should not get any opportunity to come again."

"No, no Mr. Pore, you are always welcome in our plant as an F.D.A officer and our friend."

"But not as an investigating officer." Mr. Pore diffused the tension.

All of us laughed at Mr. Pore's statement including Mr. Pore himself.

I accompanied him for lunch outside our factory.

My very first day at Boehringer Knoll was really memorable.

37

PLASTIC PILL IN A STRIP

"Manohar, can you come up in to the QC lab please?" Dr. Rajagopalan our QC Head called me.

"Yes sir. Is there any problem?"

"No, nothing serious, but I would like to discuss something with you. Please bring Shyam also with you." Shyam was my colleague and he too was a Technical Manager like myself. In fact we both shared a common room on the ground floor.

"Okay sir." I replied.

"Shyam, Dr. Raj is calling us in to his office. Come, let us go and see what the issue is."

"Okay." Shyam said, putting on his apron.

We entered the office of Dr. Rajagopalan which was attached to our QC lab. Mr. R. Sridharan was already there in the room with Dr. Raj. R. Sridharan was our Assistant QC Manager and deputy of Dr. Raj.

"Come, come have a seat." Dr. Raj told us. We sat on the two chairs in front of Dr. Raj.

"Yes sir?" Shyam and I said simultaneously.

"Manohar, see this." Dr. Raj put a strip of Septran tablet in front of us.

The strip had nine intact tablets and in one pocket, which was party opened, we could see something inside, but it was definitely not the tablet of Septran or for that matter any other tablet.

"Can I open this pocket Doctor?" I asked.

"Why not? Not only open it but see and tell me what is it". Dr. Raj said looking straight into my eyes.

"Yes sir."

I opened the pocket and I saw a small roundish plastic ball like thing, which was slightly uneven. "Looks like some plastic thing sir."

"Are you packing septran tablets or plastic balls in the strip Manohar?"

I was a little scared, and really did not know what and how to reply to Dr. Raj. Even though Dr. Raj was a friendly QC Manager but today he was not in his usual mood.

"Show me Manohar." Sridharan extended his right hand towards me. I gave him the plastic ball like thing.

"Sir, I think, Manohar and I must go down and see what must have happened there." Shyam came to my rescue.

"Not only two of you, take Sridharan along with you and report back to me."

"Yes sir." I said.

"Manohar you have to be more careful and talk to your strip machine operator also. This will damage the image of the company you know. How can we reply to the management about such things? Please go down all of you and find out what this is about." Dr. Raj softened his tone while returning to his usual mood.

We all eased out and left his room saying "Okay Sir."

All three of us came down to our room and sat down for a moment; each alternatively looking at that strange plastic ball like thing.

"Shyam, let us go to the strip sealing machine and see what this is." I said.

All three of us left the room and walked to the strip sealing machine, where three machines were strip sealing Septran tablets. We went into one of the rooms, where Sitaram Chavan, a very senior and sincere operator, was operating the machine.

"Namaskar Sir." Sitaram greeted us, "Can I help you with anything sir?" he asked.

"No, no. We just want to see the operation of this machine." I said.

"Any problem sir?"

"No, you continue with your operation, if we need anything we will ask you."

"Okay sir."

I was observing the operation and the operator both. He had a small thin knife in his hand. After every five- six minutes he used to scrape the side of the hot sealing roller with the knife to collect the extruding P.V.C from the strip, which used to come to the edge of the roller as the machine runs continuously. In between he used to take out the P.V.C with his fingers slightly roll it between his index finger and thumb and drop it in the dust bin kept at the side of the machine.

As he threw the next scrapped role of the P.V.C I picked up the dustbin and found to my surprise that many plastic ball like things similar to what we had found were there in the dustbin.

For me the mystery of the small plastic ball was resolved.

"Come Sri, Shyam we will go to our office, Sitaram can you stop the machine for a while and come with us?" I asked Sitaram.

"Yes Sir, you proceed, I will shut down the machine and come to your room sir."

"Okay."

We entered my room.

"You know Sri, what this is now?"

"Yeah, it is the scrapped P.V.C, is it not?"

"Yes it is. But now the question is how did it enter the strip." I said.

"May I come in sir?"

"Come, come Sitaram, come inside."

"Sir."

"Sitaram, we have received a market complaint."

"What is that Sir?"

"We got a piece of P.V.C in the Septran strip. See this." I showed him the strip and the plastic ball.

"How could this have gone into the strip Sitaram?" Sri asked him.

"Sir, normally it should not happen, because we drop the P.V.C beads into the dust bin."

"Then how could it happen?"

"Sir there is one possibility, when we close the machine for lunch or tea break, the roller stops and if at the same time we have a bead in our hands, in our hurry to go for tea or lunch, we may throw this down, but at times it sticks to our fingers and we try to flick it, possibly it may not fall into the dust bin but may go in the wrong way and fall on the roller or in the pocket of the roller where the tablet is supposed to fall. And if the operator overlooks then it may get sealed, when we start the machine." Sitaram explained.

"Is that the only possibility Sitaram?" I asked.

"The only other possibility is that someone has done it with malicious intention, which I don't think anyone can do."

"Okay thanks Sitaram, you can go."

"Thank you Sir." Sitaram left the room.

"Hmm. We have now got the reasons, but I don't know which is true. But I have faith in my workers; that is the only thing I can say."

We went to Dr. Raj's office and told him the probable reason. He did not express his views.

In the afternoon I called every one of my strip sealing operators, explained them the product complaint and advised them to be more careful.

I did not get any such further complaint during my stay in Burroughs.

38

MEETING THE BIG LABOUR LEADER

$\mathbf{M}$r. A. Ramachandran was Production Director of Burroughs Welcome. A really matured, seasoned and at the same time very sober and decent corporate executive.

Burroughs Welcome in 1984-85 was going through a rough labour situation. The company had one labour union and other political party labour union was trying to get entry into the company. The overall working environment was not very congenial. Labour as well as management, both sides were equally tense. Practically every day some or the other issue kept cropping up.

It was a similar day with a tense environment in the factory. The time was about three in the afternoon. I was on the ground floor in my office. My intercom rang.

"Hello, Potdar Sir, Mr. Madhukar Sarpotdar, the union leader has entered the factory. He has already gone to see our personnel manager. What shall I do?" Our security officer was on the line.

"Okay. Don't worry, I will keep Dr. Dixit and Mr. Ramachandran informed. You please go to Mr. Ramachandran's office and also take a guard with you." I gave some emergency instructions to our security chief and literally ran to Mr. Ramachandran's office. On my way

I also told Dr. Dixit, our G.M. about the same. He also joined me, and we both reached Mr. Ramachandran's office.

Mr. Madhukar Sarpotdar was a learned Personnel Manager, turned a labour unionist of a strong political party. He also had an image of a strong union leader. His party was equally well known for its massive strength and support.

Dr. Dixit was a little worried about Mr. Ramachandran, though he knew Mr. Sarpotdar.

We reached Mr. Ramachandran's office. Our security chief was also already there. He told us, "Sir, Mr. Sarpotdar is in a very bad mood and looks very angry. He has gone to our Personnel Manager's officer, where one of my deputies is present."

"Okay, okay. Don't worry." Dr. Dixit said.

We entered Mr. Ramachandran's office. He had a very big slightly roundish office. And he was sitting on his big executive chair. His table was all clean as usual. In front of him there were about six chairs.

"Yes Sudhir. What is the matter? You people look tense. Any new issue again?" Mr. Ramachandran asked Dr. Dixit in a very cool tone.

"Sir actually Mr. Sarpotdar the union leader has come and wants to meet you." Dr. Dixit spoke.

"Good. So? Sit down and we will meet him. No problem. Calm down boys." Ramachandran said and indicated us to sit down with a gesture of his hand.

While we were just sitting we heard a strong knock at the door. It could not be anyone other than Madhukar. We looked back, just as he was entering the room. Dr. Dixit got up and welcomed him.

"Good afternoon Madhukar, please come in." Dr. Dixit said to the fuming Madhukar.

"What is so good in this afternoon Dr. Dixit? I don't know." Madhukar was fuming and his face was showing the rage in his heart.

heart. I literally got scared, not only for myself but also for Mr. Ramachandran.

Ramachandran got up from his seat and came forward while extending his right hand towards Mr. Madhukar as a greeting. Mr. Madhukar hesitatingly shook hands with Mr. Ramachandran.

Ramachandran put his left hand on Mr. Madhukar's shoulder warmly.

"Madhukar, please come and have a seat here." Ramachandran said as he guided Mr. Madhukar towards a big sofa in his office room.

"Manohar, why don't you go and get some cold drinks? It is really hot this afternoon." Ramachandran asked me. I went outside the room to arrange for some cold drinks.

"Sit down Madhukar, sit down. Even if you want to discuss some hot and burning issues we can discuss these coolly. Am I right Madhu?"

Ramachandran was really a matured and magnanimous person.

We both, Dr. Dixit and I; were surprised to see the drastic change in Mr. Madhukar's behaviour. We found that he had suddenly changed and was getting back to normal. His angry face became calm and quiet.

Since Dr. Dixit knew Mr. Madhukar he took the lead to discuss the matter with him.

Meanwhile the cold drinks were served and the tense ambience climate started slowly turning into a congenial environment.

"Madhukar, Mr. Ramachandran is our factory head, Sir, Madhukar is a well-known person in his field." Dr. Dixit formally introduced them to each other.

"I can see that." Mr. Ramachandran remarked.

"Madhukar, do you have any specific issue to be discussed with Mr. Ramachandran or can we sit in my room and discuss it?" Dr. Dixit asked Madhukar.

"I think I can discuss it with you Dr. Dixit." Madhukar replied.

Both of them got up.

"I am sorry for the trouble and thanks for your really cool drink." Mr. Madhukar shook hands with Mr. Ramachandran with a soft smile on his face, which was unusual for a tough leader like him.

"My door is always open Mr. Madhukar. Anytime you have a problem feel free to come to me, always and I mean it Mr. Madhukar." Ramachandran said.

"Thank you sir." Madhukar said while leaving the office with Dr. Dixit.

I can never forget this incident. I saw once again, how a most explosive situation can be handled with maturity and sobriety. It is always a good opportunity to see how people like Ramachandran handle a tense situation and make the environment most congenial and conducive for logical discussions.

39

HIGH PERFORMANCE LIQUID CHROMATOGRAPHY

Some people are very sharp at grasping certain subjects; Mr. Ramachandran was one such person.

That day I was in Q.C. lab discussing some Q.C. issue with Mr. R. Sridharan, our assistant Q.C. Manager. Dr. Rajagopalan was on leave for a few days. Suddenly we found Mr. Ramachandran entering the lab.

"Good afternoon Sir." Sri greeted him.

"Good afternoon." He reciprocated.

"Do you want anything sir? Dr. Raj is on leave." Sri told Mr. Ramachandran.

"I know he is on leave, I have some work with you Sri."

"Yes sir."

"Sri, I will come to you after a while." I said.

"No, no Manohar, I need only five minutes with Sri, you can stay with us. Come inside." Ramachandram stopped me from leaving and we enetered the Instrument lab.

"Sri, where is your High Performance Liquid Chromatography (HPLC)?" Ramachandran asked Sri.

"Here Sir." Sri pointed towards the HPLC unit.

"Good, tell me briefly about this unit, what are its main parts, how it works, etc. Very briefly, just in five minutes."

We did not understand why he wanted to know about th HPLC and that also very briefly in just five minutes.

We knew Mr. Ramachandran was a chemical engineer and basically a production man. He was not an analyst by background. Then why did he want this information suddenly was a huge surprise to us.

Sridharan briefly told him about the HPLC parts like, columns, pump, and its functioning and role of the unit in analysis. At that time we had a "Waters" unit with us. This story dates back to nearly thirty years.

"Sir, if you want more information I will give you the operation manual of the HPLC." Sri said.

"Just show me."

Sri got the HPLC manual, Ramachandran just gave the manual a glance, flipped through a few pages and returned it to Sri.

"Thanks Sri, will you be there in the lab tomorrow?"

"Yes sir."

"I may need you. Okay thanks." Ramachandran said and left the lab.

We were trying to guess what all this meant.

Next day after lunch Sri met me near my room on the ground floor. We came to my room and sat for a while.

"Manohar you know why Ramachandran came to me yesterday?" Sri opened the talk.

"No, what for?"

"Today the "Waters" representative came to meet Mr. Ramachandran."

"So?"

"Ramachandran called me to his office."

"What for?"

"The representative wanted to discuss certain new models of "Waters" HPLC, he started talking to Mr. Ramachandran. Ramachandran listened very attentively and asked him a few questions about the HPLC columns, pumps, overall performance etc. In fact not only me, but the representative also was shocked, and answered all the queries. And then finally Mr. Ramachandran said to the representative, "good! I think you can discuss the remaining things with Mr. Sridharan, our QC Manager. Will that be okay with you?" The representative then replied, "Yes sir, thank you for your valuable time sir." And while leaving the room he added, "I am surprised sir, even with so much administrative work on your hands, you are still in touch with these technical issues of the HPLC. I am really impressed." "Yes" Ramachandran replied and we left the room"

"You know Manohar," Sri continued, "Ramachandran spent just five minutes with us yesterday and listened to me talking about the very basic things about HPLC. But today he created a very genuine impression to the "Waters" representative, as if he is a master of HPLC. Believe me the representative was both shocked and impressed. He even told me that he never expected the "Production Director" to know so much. For the Quality Head it is okay but it was not expected from the Production Director."

"Great yaar Sri. We must learn some such things from him what do you say?"

"Definitely."

The story ends here. It is not important whether Mr. Ramachandran really had indepth knowledge about HPLC or not. What is important is that he had a quest to know and a willingness to spend time and the ability to understand quickly the crux of an issue and represent the same confidently. This is definitely the quality of a good executive.

40

A Case of Simple Logic than Technology

It was an unusual day in the factory. Something or the other was going wrong since morning. I was sitting in my room with a gloomy face, Shyam was busy with his files, but occasionally looking at me. He realised that things were not good for me that day.

He got up from his chair, came in front of me and said, "What is wrong with you Manohar? Shall we go and have a cup of tea and come back? I think you need it. What do you say?"

I slowly raised my head and looked at him and said, "Come on let us go and have it."

We started walking to the corridor leading to the canteen. We had not even reached the end of the corridor where our canteen was situated, when I heard Dr. Dixit's peon calling me from behind.

"Potdar saab, Dr. Dixit is calling you to his office urgently."

We stopped and I said to Shyam, "Shyam I don't know whose face I have seen in the morning."

"Don't worry, we will go and have tea afterwards. Go now, the boss is calling you." Shyam said and I went to Dr. Dixit's cabin.

"Good morning Sir, "I greeted Dr. Dixit.

"Come, come Mr. Potdar. Meet Mr. Pradhan, our auditor from the Head Office. Pradhan, he is Mr. Potdar our Technical Manager, about whom I was talking to you. A smart young manager, he will be with you and provide any help that you may need." I was a little surprised and a little shocked by Dr. Dixit's compliment to me about being a "smart young manager". I guessed there was some difficult task ahead.

"Good morning Mr. Pradhan."

"Good morning." Mr. Pradhan reciprocated my greetings.

At the same moment the office peon entered the room with a tray of hot tea and water. He kept the tray on the table.

"Manohar, sit down and have a cup of tea and then take Mr. Pradhan to manufacturing. He wants to discuss some material productivity issues with you. When you finish the discussion we will go to lunch together. What do you say Mr. Pradhan?"

"Perfectly alright Dr. Dixit."

We had tea and left Dr. Dixit's office. We reached my office on the ground floor. The office was empty, Shyam must have been busy somewhere else. We sat down.

"Yes Mr. Pradhan tell me, what can I do for you?" I made a very formal opening.

"You can call me Sanjay, just Sanjay Mr. Potdar."

"I am Manohar. You can also call me by my first name. I would like it."

The formality vanished instantly and the entire room was filled with a congenial, friendly environment.

"Good, see Manohar, I am a chartered accountant and work with our audit department in the Head Office. Presently I am looking after plant productivity and specifically today I have come to the plant in connection with a small but very very specific issue about a product and its material productivity, which is a matter of concern." Sanjay spelled out the reason for his visit to the plant.

"Okay."

"Manohar we were going through the bulk productivity of your 20 tablet products for the last one year."

"Hmmm."

"I found that there is one product in that list which consistently shows low material productivity, that is I mean a low yield. Consistently every month this one product shows very very low yields as compared to the other products."

"I know."

"You know?"

"Yes."

"Manohar, I have gone through your monthly production reports and have read your remarks about the same, but to be frank with you I am not convinced. When all other produccts show no issues, why does only this product show a low yield every month?"

"I know, this product always showed low yield but I am also not able to put my finger on the problem yet. Sanjay, you won't believe I have checked everything more than once but all my efforts have been futile."

"I don't believe it Manohar, a man like you and your team cannot pin point the issue. I am not a chemist or a technical person but I would like to go through your manufacturing process. We may be able to find some clue, what do you say?"

"I too think so. Let me get you the product B.P.C.R (Batch Production and Control Record)"

"Good, what does this docket contain?"

"It will give you the complete process history of each batch."

"That is a good idea."

I called for the latest BPCR of the product which was just completed.

Mr. Shanbhag, my officer from the tablet department brought the file.

"Manohar, can you just once explain this to me."

"Yeah, see first there is BOM."

"What does BOM mean?"

"Bill of Materials i.e. a list of all the materials that go into the product."

"Oh I see."

"Then step wise the process is described, for example weighing, mixing, wet granulation, drying, milling, sifting, lubrication, compression and packing."

"Good!"

"At every critical step we check the weight to know the process yield."

"That's wonderful. Can I have a look at that list?"

"Why not? Please."

"I could understand only one material from this i.e. starch."

"Yes, all the others are some active and inactive substances."

"The batch size is 500 kg is it?"

"Yes, it is 500 kg."

"My god and this contains 200 kg of starch?"

"Yes this particular product has a very high starch content."

"Any specific reason for this?"

"No but the formulation is developed like that."

"Okay, okay."

Sanjay was going through the process with great interest and very carefully. He repeatedly kept looking at the yield of granulation.

"You know Manohar, you told me that you wet granulate this batch which means you make a starch paste with water and then granulate it and then dry and the granules are ready. Is it not?"

"Yes."

"And what happens to the water in the paste?"

"That gets evaporated during the drying process."

"One minute Manohar, I am only looking from the material balancing point of view. Just an arithmetic you know."

"Yes."

"See you have materials in mixing nearly 490 kg and when you mix it and dry it, that means you are adding the water and taking it out again by drying. Is it not?"

"Yes."

"That means 490 kg of material plus say five kg of water approximately you said."

"Yes."

"That means after drying that 5 kg of water will go and again you should get 490 kg."

"There will be some process loss also Sanjay."

"I agree but how much?"

"Should be about 1 to 1.5 kg."

"But Manohar I see the process loss is more than 20 kg here. Say instead of 488 kg we got only 470 kg. Is it not surprising? Where is this twenty kg material going?"

"Hmmm, you have a point Sanjay."

"You say the water is getting evaporated during the drying process, is there anything else that can be getting evaporated during the drying process?"

I relaxed on my chair, closed my eyes, put both my hands on my head and smiled with my eyes still closed.

"Hey Manohar, what happened? Are you okay?"

I opened my eyes and repeatedly thumped my fist on the table with joy.

"Sanjay, thanks yaar, thanks you very much, you are really great."

"Hey what happened suddenly, what is so great about me? At least tell me."

"Sanjay you solved the mystery of the low yield for me."

"Tell me yaar."

"Listen we are using 200 kg of starch in this batch."

"This starch contains about 10-12 % of moisture in it i.e. water. That means there is already about 20 kg of water in the material. We use two hundred kg of hydrated starch means we actually use only 180 kg of starch with nearly 20 kg water in it. The final product has only about 1.5-2 % moisture. This means nearly 18 kg of moisture is getting evaporated during our drying process and that is why we are always getting a low yield after drying, because this water gets lost in the drying process. That means that it is not the process loss but it is the loss of water, we only need to adjust the amount of starch as the amount of dried starch. Then there is only a normal process loss which may be around 1.5-2%. Thanks again."

"That's good. Then my job is done."

"And mine too. I did not understand this silly thing that we have overlooked all these days."

"Manohar, there was no pharmacy or chemistry in this issue it was only logic."

"I agree with you Sanjay. Come let us enjoy our lunch with Dr. Dixit."

We left our room and went to join Dr. Dixit for lunch.

41

FREE TRIP TO LONDON

Burrough Wellcome plant in Mumbai used to be audited by its parent auditors regularly. Normally it used to be audited once a year, and sometimes more often. Usually Mr. Mike How who was the auditor used to visit our Mumbai plant along with his team. Mr. Shyam Khante the other Technical Manager and I used to accompany him in his plant audit activities, and report the finding to Dr. S.M Dixit and Mr. A. Ramachandran. Dr. Rajagopalan and R. Sridharan also used to join us as and when the need arose.

Once we were discussing the M.P.C.Rs (Master Production and Control Records) of some of the products of tablet manufacturing, and we were talking about the possibility of variations in the output, even using the same M.P.C.R procedures. This statement of ours was challenged by Mr. Mike, the Chief Technical Auditor. He was firm and confident in his statement that if the product procedure was followed exactly then no variations can take place in the final product.

When we all were in a light mood, Mr. Mike gave us an offer, he said, "Manohar, I give you an offer. You monitor 5 batches of septran following the exact same procedure and if any one parameter varies beyond the specifications I will lose anything."

"Anything?" I asked.

"Okay I will give you a £100" Mike said.

He was there for ten days. I monitored 5 batches of Septran, but no batch showed variation beyond the specification.

We were the ones who lost. Not Mike. How did that happen?

On the tenth day, that is on the day that Mike was to return to U.K, we were having a cup of tea in Dr. Dixit's chamber.

"Manohar, today I extend you my offer again."

"What is that offer Mike?" I asked.

"See, you have to follow the exact procedure and show me the batch failing, let it be any product, tablet, liquid, injection, anything."

"And suppose it fails?"

"I will give you a free London ticket and cover all your expenses throughout your stay in London. Will you accept? I am not expecting anything in return from you, okay?"

"I will try. I accept your bet. Do you agree or do you want to back out?"

"No! No way!" Mike confirmed.

Mr. Mike left for London. I was there for nearly three years as the Technical Manager (Manufacturing). I was waiting for a London trip but "fortunately" I never got a free trip to U.K., during my stay.

The story ends here. This was to show how much confidence Mike had in the manufacturing procedure.

42

A Good Fishy Smell

We used to use lot of glycerine in our liquid formulations. Once we received a very big consignment from U.K.

One of the tests for glycerine involved taking about 10 ml of glycerine in a test tube, warming it slightly and then smelling the vapours that come out from the glycerine. The acceptable observation should be "Agreeable smell."

The sample was given to a chemist who was analysing it for the first time, and incidentally a strict vegetarian.

He took 10 ml of the sample and warmed it in a test tube and smelled it. The smell was so strong he could not bear it. According to him the smell was very bad. He reported the remark in his work book as "The smell is very bad, dirty, nauseating, offensive, etc. and hence the product/ batch stands rejected."

He did not perform any of the other tests and gave the report to Shridharan. Shridharan advised him to carry out all the other tests as well and then submit the report.

He did that and then reported that the batch was passing all the other tests perfectly. The matter went to Dr. Rajagopalan, he was not in a position to decide immediately. He said, "Sri, ask somebody to repeat that "Smell" test only."

Shridharan gave the test to Dr. Zachary D'souza, our chief microbiologist.

He performed the test and reported as follows, "it has a good fishy smell. Product acceptable." Incidentally Dr. Zach was from Goa and liked sea food.

Now Dr. Rajgopalan was in a fix over which report to accept. Meanwhile Mr. Peter Cook entered the room where we were sitting and discussing about the glycerine issue. Peter Cook was an analyst from U.K. on a visit to India.

He asked, "What is the issue Raj?"

Dr. Rajgopalan explained to him the whole story and also requested him to give his opinion about the matter.

Peter Cook performed the test and came back to the office and said, "the smell is normal, agreeable, no issues. It passes the test perfectly."

We were in a funny situation. The three reports were,

- "The smell is bad, dirty, offensive, etc."
- "The smell is good fishy." And
- "The smell is normal and agreeable."

The reports were influenced by the analyst's background.

Finally the product was accepted by taking into consideration Peter Cook's report which was "The smell is normal and agreeable."

43

MISBRANDED DRUG

Those were the days when we used to get a lot of complaints about misbranded Septran tablets from the market. Some of these drugs were with names that were similar sounding and similarly spelt to Septran, like Septram, Saptran, etc.

One day Dr. Rajgopalan called me to his room upstairs.

When I entered his room, he was sitting with Shridharan and on his table I found a box (carton) of Septran tablets.

"Come, come Manohar. You have a gift again." Raj made a light hearted remark.

"What is the news today sir?" I asked.

"Misbranded Septran again." Raj said.

I sat on the chair and looked at the strips from the carton.

"Have you got the analyst's report from the lab sir?" I asked and then continued further, "These strips look exactly like ours, we must check the assays."

"No need Manohar, I am one hundred percent sure that the tablets will fail in the assay, because they are not our strips."

"How can you be so confident sir, that even without analysing the tablets, you can say that they are not ours?"

"By physical observation Manohar."

"What physical observation? You have not even opened the strips." I said in surprise.

"Manohar, see the over printing details on the strip."

I took a closer look.

"They are okay, price, batch number, all other over printing details match Sir." I said.

"No they are not matching." Dr. Raj showed me another carton of the same batch. "Now see and tell me, what is the difference?" I looked at both the strips and was not able to find any difference.

"They look the same to me sir."

"Manohar, you are a production guy, you cannot observe this."

"What is that which I can't see sir?"

"Manohar, see the "QUALITY" of the over printing."

I observed very carefully, one strip was showing slightly smudged printing while the other was perfectly clear.

"Yes, one has smudged printing and the other is clear." I said.

"Now you got it. You know the smudged printing is our genuine product and the one with the clear printing is misbranded. The misbranded product collected from the market shows a very high quality printing, much much better than our product."

I had no answer. I kept quiet for a moment and then said, "Yes, it is."

"The lesson to us is we need to improve our quality of printing, quality of product alone is not enough." Dr. Raj said in a jovial manner.

"I agree with you Sir, and assure you that we will improve the quality of over printing."

44

DOUBLE BATCH NUMBERING

Controlling manufacturing process in the plant is always a tricky process. Manufacturing pharmacists are always in a hurry to proceed with the manufacturing and by typical mental frame of a manufacturing oriented person, he always hates to wait for the Q.C./Q.A./I.P.Q.C. results even if they are delayed for genuine reasons.

The Q.C./ I.P.Q.C people find it difficult to stop the manufacturing process till they are ready with their analytical results.

There is a normal process of starting primary packaging activities only after the bulk release is received by packaging from Q.C. lab. In BurroughsWellcome (as with many other companies) the packaging pharmacists are always in a hurry to start primary packaging and used to get uncomfortable if the release of the bulk was delayed. And at the time they used to start the packaging even before they receive the bulk release report. (based on their trend of reports and personal confidence). This in fact is a totally wrong practice and needed to be stopped in the interest of the company.

The Q.C department thought a lot about this and finally decided on a system to control this practice, which did work well.

The system was like this: the bulk manufacturing starts with a "provisional batch number." This will be used till the bulk batch is manufactured and bulk sample collected by the I.P.Q.C for testing.

Once the bulk batch is tested and if it is released for packaging then the batch will be assigned the "Permanent batch number" or "Final batch number". This batch number is required to be printed on the primary packs like labels, cartons, strips, etc.

Due to this system, you cannot start primary packaging because you cannot over print the batch number on the primary or other packaging materials.

In my opinion this system can be applied in practically all companies, to ensure a proper control on the packaging operation i.e. packaging should start only after the bulk product is released.

45

GMP - DAY

After eighteen years of industrial experience in multination pharmaceutical organisations like Hoechst, Boehringer Knoll, Burroughs Well come, etc., on 25th January, 1987, I joined a leading Indian Pharmaceutical organisation as Manufacturing Manger. The H.R.D Manager took me around the plant for about 2 hours and finally he brought me to the central packaging department and introduced me to the central packaging department Manager. He asked me, "Sir, how do you find the plant?" I replied, "It is very good, neat, clean and tidy." I said, "I am impressed, but I find only one thing amazing. There was very low activity in all the departments. Is it because it is the last week of the month and you have practically finished your production schedule of the month?" The Manager replied in innocence, "No sir, it is because today we are celebrating the GMP day."

"What do you mean by that?" I asked.

"Sir, today we follow GMP in the plant."

"And what do you do on the other days?"

"Production sir." Was the reply of the Manager.

I was surprised by his answer but I still continued the conversation. I asked, "But why don't you follow GMP on all the days?" The

Manager replied with complete innocence again, "Sir, if we follow GMP on all days, then when will we do the production?"

I was amazed by his answer. Believe me, the above incident and conversation is one hundred percent true. And this incident is deeply carved in my mind for ever. Remember this was the concept about GMP, not only in that company but in many companies twenty five years back, in India.

46

LEARNING FROM Mr. PARAB OF LUPIN

I joined Lupin Laboratories in 1987 as Manufacturing Manager. Before that, whichever companies I worked in, I had never manufactured a single batch of sugar coated tablet myself. At that time sugar coating was a very popular technique used in the pharmaceutical manufacturing (film coating had not become so popular at that time). Secondly, the coating operations were carried out by using simple open pan coating followed by wax polishing. Auto coaters etc. were not available in many companies.

We had a few products in this class of coated tablets. Somehow I wanted to learn this technique myself.

We had Mr. Vaman Parab, as an expert sugar coater with us. I decided to talk to him. One day I entered the tablet coating section where Vaman was coating a batch.

"Vaman which product are you coating today?" I asked.

He named the product.

"When is this batch getting over?"

"By 4:00 P.M. Sir."

"Okay, see, when you start the next batch tell me. Don't start anything before you tell me."

"Any problem sir?"

"No, no problem, I just want to learn tablet coating from you, I will be working with you for one full batch of the next product. And you will be teaching me the entire process that is involved. Will you?" I asked him.

"Sir are you kidding?"

"No Vaman I am not, I really want to learn from you. I hope you don't mind."

"I will be embarrassed Sir, you are the manufacturing Manager and I am just an operator. How can I teach you?"

"Don't worry I know you know the process and you have skill. I know the theory of the coating process but I have not coated any batch myself and hence I lack the skill, which you have, and I want to learn. Please don't get embarrassed, I am going to do exactly as you tell me and show me. Okay? I will come tomorrow morning and work with you?" I said.

"Okay Sir. I will show you everything." Vaman promised me.

The next two days I literally worked with Vaman, no sorry, not with him, under his tutelage. In those two days I practiced everything related to sugar coating of tablets.

I know for certain, coating of a single batch of tablets will not make me an expert coater like Vaman, but I definitely experienced the thrill of coating a batch.

I thanked Mr. Vaman Parab for his teaching.

I narrated this story only to emphasize to the young manufacturing pharmacists that they have to learn practically every manufacturing skill from the workers to back up your theoretical background. Only then you will become a real manufacturing pharmacist.

When I was working with Hoechst, we were told that we must acquire every skill that our operators have in our section, even though we may not always be required to use them.

47

ASKING QUESTIONS

I always tell my students in class to please ask questions, make the life of your teachers miserable by asking appropriate questions so that you will also learn and your teachers will continue to study.

All through school and college education we are taught to answer questions which somebody will ask us, whether it is in the classroom or in the examination hall.

I learnt this myself for the first time in Lupin.

We were to go for a computerised production planning and control system. Company had hired a software development agency to make a P.P.C system for our Aurangabad operations. Mr. P.V. Bhandarkar, Works Manager, organised a small committee, consisting of;

- Mr. P.V. Bhandarkar – Chairperson
- Mr. Anil Gupta – PPC Manager
- Mr. Pabitro Chattarjee – Production Manager and
- Myself – Manufacturing Manager

We had our first meeting in Mr. P.V Bhandarkar's office with the software developer. The software developer explained the objective and scope of his consultancy. At the end he said,

"We have a starting point, i.e., a production plan and an end point as delivering of the finished products to the finished goods and then executing the distribution of the finished goods. Am I right?"

"Yes" Said Mr. Bhandarkar.

"Now as I understand from Mr. Anil and Dr. Potdar you have a number of steps in this process starting from receiving a production plan to distribution of the finished products where required."

"Correct." said Mr. Bhandarkar.

"Mr. Bhandarkar, now I want from you a list, a really really long list of questions, may be something around a hundred questions or one fifty or even more if you can."

"What questions?" Anil and I asked simultaneously.

"Yeah I will tell you. Imagine all the possible questions in this process of manufacturing that will be asked by your colleagues, your bosses, your subordinates, etc. "

"We did not get your point" Mr. Bhandarkar said.

The consultant explained – "See, for example you are the factory head and your boss is sitting in Mumbai Head Office and he wants to know,

1. What is the volume of production this month?
2. What is the capacity utilization of the tablet department?
3. Which materials are short for the months production?
4. Will you be running over time or in shift this month?
5. When will Nigeria export order no. N 316 be executed?

Or anything like these. Remember the questions will not only be from your boss but from your colleagues and subordinates also." he explained.

"But there will be so many questions, how do we list all of them?" I asked.

He suggested a simple way, "Go very very systematically."

"What does that mean?" I asked him again.

"First list various steps in the manufacturing process, then list various levels of people, starting right from the worker to vice-president sitting in your Mumbai office, you know.

"Okay."

"Then from each level and activity generate possible interactions and from these interactions you will be able to generate questions for which you should have answers. It is my job to study your questions and show you how these questions will be answered using my system, which I will develop."

"Oh my god! this is a herculean task."

"I know, but it can be done easily if we work very systematically."

 With this the meeting concluded.

For nearly the entire next week, Anil and I worked on identifying questions. It was definitely a herculean task. The list became very big like Hanuman's tail. The number exceeded more than 150 questions to start with.

In the next meeting we showed this list to the consultant. He said, "My task is now simple because of these 150 questions."

"What do you mean?" I asked.

"Dr. Potdar, when we go through each of these questions we are actually going to identify many more questions."

"Don't tell me." I said.

"Don't worry rest of the work I will do and come to you after a few days."

The process went on through a couple of meetings and finally we got our computerised "Production Planning and Control System."

The lesson from this was "asking questions is more difficult than answering them. The only condition necessary is that the questions should be appropriate."

So develop a good habit of asking appropriate questions.

48

WORKING FOR PEOPLE

Normally when we answer a question like, "for whom you are working?" We answer by saying, "I work for Lupin or I work for Cadila etc." which is perfectly normal. But is that the right answer? May be. But I personally feel the still more appropriate answer is "I work for Mr. Bhandarkar or I work for Mr. Agarwal etc."

I have been lucky enough to meet people like Dr. J. G. Bhat (Q.C Head of M.S.D.), Dr Ravi Rosha of Hoechst, Mr. Bhandarkar of Lupin, Mr. A.K Agarwal of Ranbaxy and Lupin, Mr. V.P. Samant of Boehringer Knoll, Mr. S.N Desai of Cadila, Mr. Bhaskar Patel (M.D. of Plethico), Raghuvir Mangalurkar; General Manager of CFL, Goa. All these people had totally different character but one thing in common, that was, a pro-employee attitude and an ability to take people together and lead from the front.

Mr. P.V Bhandarkar of Lupin, at that time Works Manager of Lupin Aurangabad plant was head of the factory. I am not exaggerating when I claim that he practically knew every person in the plant, both officers and workmen together, by their names. It is really not by virtue of his memory power but by virtue of his personal interest in every person who was working in his factory.

When anyone invited him to any function at their homes, he would always turn up there for at least a little while, be it the house of an officer or a workman.

Without fail he would greet every officer and above on their birthday, believe me, he was not doing it as a formality but from deep within his heart.

I realised this for the first time when I was handling an important export order and we had a very short time to meet the deadline.

I called a meeting of my concerned officers, key operators from manufacturing and packaging, and the Production Manager Mr. Pabitro Chatterjee. I discussed the work plan and told them that the time is short and the order is prestigious. I said, "It is a challenge and we must succeed." I also delivered a sort of motivating speech to this group.

Everyone was listening to what I was saying. At the end one very senior operator got up and said, "Sir you don't worry, we will meet the challenge and see that the export order is executed in time. We assure you sir." I was very happy; I thought my dialogue and speech had worked. But I realised a moment later that this was not the sole effect of my speech, when I heard the operator told me at the end of his sentence, "Sir, we will not ever let down Mr. Bhandarkar. 'Bhandarkar Saranchya ibraticha prashna ahe' (It is a question of Mr. Bhandarkar's prestige.)"

After so many years I still remember that small incident and the warm feeling these workmen had for Mr. Bhandarkar.

The reason for this was very simple. Mr. Bhandarkar sincerely cared for his people and they reciprocated the same.

49

AVOID GROSS CONTAMINATION

This is a story of status and understanding of cGMP twenty five years ago. I had recently joined an Indian Pharmaceutical company as the Head of the manufacturing department. My boss, the works Manager of the company put me on 10 days induction programme.

I was going through all the departments, section by section and observing the activities each section was carrying out and how.

I entered the tablet granulation section, the area was titled as "Granulation Hall" i.e. the name plate on that section. Inside the section there were three conventional mixers cum granulators, they were open type. There was only one senior operator and a pharmacist in that area.

"Good morning Sir." The pharmacist greeted me.

"Good morning, what is going on today in your section?" I asked.

"Granulation sir."

"Good, which product and which batches?"

He named the product and also told me which batches.

"Are you manufacturing three different products in the same room?" I asked in surprise and worry which was clearly visible on my face. (Please keep in mind that I had worked about 16 years in a multinational company before joining this company.)

"Sir, three products in three different mixers sir." He explained.

"Yes I can see that. Anyway you cannot granulate three different products in one granulator at the same time. Right?"

"Yes sir."

I further checked and saw that the room had only one Air Handling Unit.

"Okay. Proceed with your work."

"Okay Sir." The pharmacist replied and continued his work with his operator.

I was just observing their operations without making any comments. I saw the operator was going from one granulator to another, putting his hand in the granulator, taking some material from it pressing it in his palms and again breaking the material and dropping it in the same granulator, then going to the next granulator and repeating the same. He was trying to see whether the granulation was complete or not, so that he can take up the material for sieving and then drying etc. He was cleaning his hand just by rubbing it on his boiler suit on his hip. He did not think that he was doing anything wrong, neither did the pharmacist. Only I was shocked and was literally getting scared.

I left the section and went to my boss's office. He was sitting in his chair, looking at some papers on his table.

"Good morning sir." I greeted him.

"Good morning, good morning, come, come, have a seat." He welcomed me and pushed a switch for a bell. The bell rang outside and the office peon came into the room.

I sat on the chair in front of him as he ordered two cups of tea.

"Tell me Manohar, how is your induction going on?" he started the conversation.

"Good." I gave a short reply.

"Sir I see a serious problem in the tablet granulation section." I started telling him the scene in the tablet granulation room. I continued, "Sir, there are tremendous chances of cross contamination in the product because we have three granulators, one A.H.U and one operator. It is very serious and we need to do something about it urgently to avoid the chances of cross contamination in this area." I put forward my concern about the manufacturing practices being followed.

"I know, Manohar, but you need not be so worried about 'Cross contamination'. See that there is no 'Gross contamination'." He replied in an absolutely unperturbed manner.

The term 'gross contamination' was new for me. In fact I had never heard of it before. I got confused.

"What do you mean by 'Gross contamination' Sir?," was my most innocent question to him.

"Simple, see that the operator is not adding say; Ibuprofen instead of Paracetamol, this is very serious you know. This has to be avoided at any cost. We just cannot accept this. this is what I call 'gross contamination'."

I was shocked at his reply but seriously scared also.

This was the cGMP environment, not only in that company but in many other companies as well. Thanks to the efforts of the Pharmaceutical industry and F.D.A. too, in the last twenty five years, the cGMP scenario has totally changed from what it was at that time to what it is presently.

The company today has approvals from most international auditors like USFDA, MHRA etc.

50

MANAGERIAL STYLE

I joined Cadila Laboratories Limited in the year 1990 as "Production controller" in their Ahmedabad plant at Ghodasar.

I was responsible for the production activities of the plant and was reporting to Mr. Suryakant N. Desai, who was V.P (Technical) and also my boss.

I observed a few things about him, which I found would be useful to any manager and I adopted it in my practice as well.

First thing I had observed was that, he used to be the first person to enter the plant in the general shift and the last person to leave the plant.

In 1990's there was no C.C.T.V coverage of the entire plant, wherein the boss can see everything sitting in his chamber. Mr. Desai used to come to his room put on his apron, put a small notebook and pen in his apron pocket and leave the room for a round of the plant. He would start from the warehouse and then move through all the sections of the manufacturing, engineering, etc. finally he would come to the Q.C lab which was on the first floor, where his office was also located.

He would meet each of the section managers after the entire round of the section and ask them if they had any issues to be discussed with him and he would also discuss anything that was worth mentioning, incidences or adverse observations he has made during the visit.

He used to note down certain things in his small pocket note book. He used to take about one and a half to two hours every day to do this and then come to his room, remove his apron, relax a bit and maybe order a cup of tea.

Based on the things he wrote in his notebook, he would call the concerned people and talk to them about his observation, give instructions etc. or ask for some information.

His style used to keep him constantly informed about the plant activities. He used to have a pulse of the working of the plant. He practically used to meet all the section level people and have a dialogue with them, and more important he maintained a personal contact with not only officers and managers but also many of the workers. This used to help him taking the entire team along with him for the benefit of the organisation.

I learnt a lot from his style and adopted the same in my career as a Senior Manager.

51

Dr. WILLOW'S INSPECTION

It was the year 1992 or 1993; I was Plant Manager of 'Ranbaxy' at Dewas in Madhya Pradesh.

That time we had 2 pharma plants at Dewas, they were called Plant- A and Plant –B. Plant- A was also called SSP (Semi Synthetic Penicillin Plant) and Plant –B was called NAB (Non Anti biotic Plant) and the third plant was to come up shorty, Plant –C; Cephalosporin Plant.

We were planning for the third upcoming plant for M.C.A approval (now M.H.R.A). One consultant from U.K had come to Dewas, by name Dr. Willows. He was advising us on the MHRA requirements and preparing us for the same. (MCA was earlier called as Department of Health and Social Security)

Mr. Willows first came to Delhi and from there he reached Dewas. He was sitting in Mr. A.K. Agarwals office on the first floor. Mr. A.K. Agarwal was the plant controller of Dewas i.e. he was heading the entire Dewas operations.

When I entered Mr. Agarwal's office, they were having tea, "Good morning Mr. Agarwal." I greeted my boss. "Good morning, come meet Dr. Willows from UK. He is our cGMP advisor for upcoming DHSS approval. Dr. Willows, Mr. Potdar is our Plant Manager, looking after manufacturing activities."

"Good morning Dr. Potdar." Willows said.

"Good morning Sir."

"Sit down Manohar, sit down." Mr. Agarwal said. I occupied the chair next to Dr. Willows. "Manohar, Mr. Willows wants visit both our plants A and B with you."

"Not only with Dr. Potdar, Mr. Agarwal you will also accompany us." Dr. Willows corrected Mr. Agarwal.

"Yes of course, all three of us will go round the plants." Mr. Agarwal corrected himself.

"Mr. Agarwal, can I go to the plant? When you are ready tell me I will join you." I said.

"No, no, Dr. Potdar please you are not going anywhere. Now we are ready, let me finish off the last sip of tea and then we can get moving." Dr. Willows stopped me.

Both Mr. Agarwal and I looked at each other with a somewhat suspicious thought in our minds.

"Come on Mr. Agarwal, let us take a round of your facilities." Dr. Willows said as he put his cup down after finishing the last sip of tea.

A new apron was already arranged for Dr. Willows. We left Mr. Agarwal's room while Dr. Willows was still putting his apron on. We reached the staircase and started walking down to come out of the main administrative building to go to our Plant – A

"Now please listen to me, my friends." Dr. Willows addressed us in a typical English style.

"Sir." I said.

"When we move through the plant, no one, I mean no one will speak anything. We will just move from section to section, both of you and I too, will only observe, what and how things are going on?"

"Okay." agreed Mr. Agarwal nodding his head in approval.

"It seems you have a beautiful rose garden in the plant Mr. Agarwal." Willows remarked pleasantly while looking at the left side of the road where we had a really beautiful rose garden. Thanks to our chief security officer, Captain Naresh; a young, dynamic, very fair and smart ex-army officer and his gardening team.

"Sir, people generally say we have a garden in the plant but in fact we have the plant in the garden, because what you see is only a small part of the rose gardens in our plant." I said. He looked at me with his eyebrows raised, but I noticed a notorious smile on his face.

"Wonderful, you are right doctor." Dr. Willows said.

"So, coming back to the point," Willows cut short the appreciation of the garden and quickly came back to the point of discussion.

"We will not talk anything, we will only observe, is that clear gentlemen?"

"Yes sir." I confirmed.

"Whatever we want to talk and discuss, we will do it in Mr. Agarwal's office when we go back. Okay?"

"Yes sir."

We arrived at plant A's gate came and took a right turn to enter the plant. On the right side was the room of Mr. Sunil Singhai, the Production Manager of plant – A, we entered his room. He was looking at some paper on his table.

"Good morning Sunil." I greeted him.

"Good morning." He got up from his chair as he looked to Mr. Agarwal and an elderly matured white man with us.

"Sunil, he is Dr. Willows our UK consultant. He is Mr. Sunil Singhai, Plant – A Production Manager."

"Good morning, young man."

"Good morning sir."

"Sunil, Dr. Willows wants to see your plant, in fact all of us will be going on this round, from section to section, starting from raw material receiving bay, till the end of our finishing section." I told Sunil. Sunil reached for his telephone on the table by his right hand, probably he wanted to alert his people in the plant that, be careful, someone is coming inside.

"Don't Mr. Sunil, don't use your telephone for some time." Willows said while patting his hand on the telephone receiver preventing Sunil from making any call.

"Shall we move to the plant Mr. Agarwal?" Dr. Willows asked.

"Sunil, Dr. Willows wants that during the visit none of us speak anything, we are only going to observe what and how things are going on in the plant, and any talk, discussion, etc. we will have in Mr. Agarwal's cabin after the plant round." I cleared the premise.

"Yes." Dr. Willows nodded his head in approval.

For the next hour or so we were moving from section to section in Plant – A. Dr. Willows was carefully observing the situations, activities, people, materials, machines, cleaning of the facility, uniforms of the people, the way they work, their behaviour, their actions and everything. This was a totally new approach for all of us i.e. see, only see but control yourself from saying anything. It was really unbearable; none of us were tuned to such a plant visit or a so called audit. We were in an altogether different tense environment. We looked at many unacceptable, wrong, undesirable things, but did not utter a single word. You can imagine the tension laden silent tour. Finally we completed the tour of the plant. We rested for a while in Sunil's room to have a glass of water and then left plant- A along with Sunil and went to Mr. Agarwal's room.

Mr. Willows and Mr. Agarwal entered the room, I asked Sunil to arrange for some tea and then join us.

"Haha, what a hectic tour Mr. Willows" Mr. Agarwal spoke in a relaxing tone. 'I never had such a silent plant visit." Mr. Agarwal added.

"Okay. Let me say a few things first and then you can comment upon it. Is that okay?" Dr. Willows asked.

"Perfectly alright sir." Mr. Agarwal said while revolving a bit in his chair.

"See Mr. Agarwal I stopped Dr. Potdar from going to the plant before our visit and also Mr. Sunil from calling his plant people on the phone before we entered the plant. Am I right?"

"Yes sir." Mr. Agarwal said while we were looking at Mr. Willows face with a big question mark clearly visible on our faces.

"Do you know the reason Mr. Agarwal?"

"Why?"

"I wanted to see and observe and make my own impression about your Plant – A in the most natural working environment, without any window dressing. What we have observed in the last one hour in your plant is what happens every day. Am I right?"

"Yes sir."

"There are many observations I have made in the last one hour; it made a certain first hand impression on me as an auditor. I will give you a written report on this tomorrow."

"Okay." I said.

"You as production Manager, Plant Manager and Plant Controller look at that report tomorrow and maybe after a day or so give me your individual comments about that report. Please do not discuss your comments amongst yourselves till then. What I am doing is all and only in the interest of your Plant."

"I am not a police man and my report is not going to be an investigation report, no not in any way. They are my friendly observations for our benefit, and when I say 'our' I am included too, because from now onwards until the D.H.S.S approval I am a member of your team and the success in the D.H.S.S. approval is going to be "our success". I have worked with D.H.S.S for a long time and hence I know what D.H.S.S. looks for. My association with you will help us to achieve our common objective. This is what I not only think but know for certain."

Mr. Willows took a pause. His simple talk changed the entire environment, which was really tensed earlier but had become much more relaxed now.

The peon got the tea and biscuits on a tray which he kept on the table. He opened a bottle of mineral water, poured into fresh clean glasses and left the room.

"Relax boys, relax." Willows said looking at Sunil and me.

"Thank you sir." I replied.

"Mr. Agarwal , anyway you will receive my detailed report tomorrow but while having a cup of tea I would like to talk about a small observation in today's plant visit." He continued his narration while having his first sip of the hot tea. "Remember when we entered the tablet coating section of your tablet department; the operator was busy with his work and was doing something in the rotating coating pan. (At that time we did have the conventional coating pans also). As we entered, the operator got a little shocked looking at us; three of his senior managers with a "white man" suddenly entering the work place. Probably he got a little scared also. I am sure. Because of this suddenness, I saw some tablets from his hand fallen down on the ground, which he quickly picked up by hand and placed both his hands behind his back. The tablets which he had collected were in the palms of his right hand. All the while we were in the room he was facing us with his hand behind his back. Then when we left the room I wanted to go back and see what he had done with the tablets in his hand. But I did not go, my more than forty years of experience tells me that the moment we left the room, he must have put those tablets which he had picked up from the ground into the tablet pan which was coating the tablet."

"Probably you are right Mr. Willows." Mr. Agarwal accepted the fact reluctantly.

"If he has not done that, I would be the most happiest person in the world." Willow continued, "But the chances are less."

Sunil and I were silent listeners to what Dr. Willows was saying. We knew for certain that what he was saying was the truth.

"What is important here Mr. Agarwal is that when you coat millions of tablets following the current technology, some tablets are definitely going to fall on the ground. Nothing wrong with that, nothing you can do to avoid this. But what is important is, the operator should know what to do about the tablets that have fallen on the ground. How will he know? He must be trained. Trained; Mr. Agarwal." Willow said.

"Yes Dr. Willows, you are right." Mr. Agarwal agreed and we nodded our heads.

"Dr. Potdar and Sunil, it is primarily your duty to see that, you have Standard Operating Procedures (SOPs) that are not a mere decoration but are actually practiced, and this is only possible if you tell them what to do and 'WHY'?" Dr. Willows emphasised by stressing the word "WHY?"

"You are right sir. We will see that all our workmen not only understand the Standard Operating Procedures (SOPs) but also practice them and know the "WHY" behind every activity they do." I assured Dr. Willows.

"Good, thank you. I will meet you people tomorrow. You can now go back to your plant. Let me spend some time with Mr. Agarwal here."

"Thank you Sir." I said as Sunil and I left Mr. Agarwal's office. On the way back to our office we were mentally preparing about how to proceed with training the workmen.

52

BACKLOG OF INCOMPLETE BPCRs

In the year 1991, I joined Ranbaxy Dewas as Plant Manager. The Ranbaxy facility was having two pharmaceutical plants A and B and a third facility C was to come up soon. There was another plant manufacturing bandages.

Mr. Agarwal was the Plant Controller i.e., the Head of the Location. Each plant had a Production Manager and a Plant Manager to look after all the plants.

When I joined the factory Mr. Agarwal said to me, "Manohar, I see that our BPCRs (Batch Production and Control Records) are not up-to-date in both the plants and I want you to see what the exact status is and how we can keep them up-to-date."

"Okay sir, I will first review the status and then come back to you to report on any corrective action needed." I said.

I had two senior Production Managers in the plant, I discussed it with them and working together with each of the Production Manager, we found out how many BPCRs are incomplete and to what extent and if we need to complete them how much manpower and time will be needed.

I collected the basic data and went to Mr. Agarwal and said, "Sir I have gone through the BPCRs and I found out that a little more than one hundred BPCRs are incomplete in some way or the other, in both plants put together i.e., Plant – A and Plant – B. I have not looked into the bandage manufacturing plant since that plant is not under my control."

"Okay, so what is your plan to complete this and update all the BPCRs in every respect?" Mr. Agarwal looked at me.

"We can work extra hours for say about fifteen days in both plants and complete the task sir. I have also discussed this plan with our Q.C Manager Mr. Uma Nandan. He too is very concerned about this issue."

"That is one way, but I have a different idea in mind for this task."

"What is that sir?"

"See Manohar, we have second and fourth Saturday off. I think next Saturday is second Saturday. We will call all the pharmacists and managers on that Saturday and Sunday and get all the BPCRs updated. I will call Mr. Uma Nandan and some of his Q.C persons also to complete the work. What do you say?"

"I think we should discuss this with our Production Managers and finalise the plan."

"Good, you call Sunil, Ramesh and Uma Nandan also to my room. I want to thrash out this matter immediately." Sunil and Ramesh were the Prouction Managers of our Plant A and B respectively.

We had a meeting in Mr. Agarwals office. He explained the seriousness of the incomplete BPCRs and told them that he wanted all the incomplete BPCRs to be updated in these two days.

Everyone agreed.

That second Saturday and Sunday practically every supervisory and managerial staff reported for duty and the completion of the BPCRs task was done on a war footing.

On Monday Mr. Agarwal called Sunil, Ramesh, Uma Nandan and me and said, "I am happy that the job is over but now onwards don't keep anything pending like this, and Uma Nandan you are not going to release any batch under any circumstances if the BPCR of that batch is not submitted to you in the completed form. Is that clear to you all?"

"Yes sir." we all said.

After that we did not have any problem in this regard.

53

I DON'T WANT TO SEE YOUR FACES

Mr. Pushpender Singh Bindra was our new Location Head of Ranbaxy at the time of our first MCA approval of Dewas pharamaceutical plant –C i.e. Cephalosporin plant. Mr. Sunil Singhai was transferred to this plant as Production Manager from his Plant – A.

The plant – C was a newly constructed facility and was under validation. The MCA inspection of this plant was after about six months.

Mr. Bindra was a mechanical engineer by education and a tough administrator and a perfect disciplinarian. He told all the concerned people that he wanted the plant to be approved in the first inspection itself. He would not accept any failure. Sometimes he jocularly used to say if we get the approval in the first instance, you will have a feather in your cap, but if you don't, I will have a cap of your feathers. Though it was a joke, the message was very loud and clear.

Everybody worked day and night like there was no tomorrow. Finally the date for the inspection came. The inspection was for three days. Last one week before the inspection was really hectic. The last two days before inspection many of us stayed in the plant overnight.

The two days of inspection were also very gruelling. Everybody put in their best during those days. On the third day of inspection, in the post lunch session, the chief inspector of M.C.A told Mr. Bindra, "Your plant is approved. I will send the official report to you when I reach back to UK."

Mr. Bindra communicated the result of the inspection to the plant. Everyone was in a joyous mood. Bindra declared a party in the evening to all the concerned people of the plant. The party was arranged in a hotel in Indore. It went on literally till midnight and that night we saw a completely different side of Mr. Bindra.

Next day the plant started as usual and I was sitting in my room as the intercom rang, "Hello."

"Manohar, please come to my room." Mr. Bindra was on the line.

I went to his office and saw that Mr. Agarwal was already there.

"Good morning sir." I greeted both of them.

"Good morning. Manohar you have the list of the ten-fifteen people who worked tirelessly for the M.C.A approval, I want all of them here immediately." Mr. Bindra said.

"Any problem sir." I asked.

"You call them first and then I will tell you what the problem is."

I was a little worried. Till yesterday everything was alright. I could not understand what happened overnight. I was unable to guess.

Within the next fifteen minutes all the officers were there in the office.

"We will go to the conference room, come on all of you." Mr. Bindra said.

Everyone was little scared.

"Sit down all of you."

The atmosphere was very tense.

"As you know," Mr. Bindra started addressing, "we have got the MCA approval for our new Cephalosporin plant."

"Yes sir." was the response from the group.

Mr. Bindra took a long pause.

"Now listen to me." All eyes turned to Mr. Bindra.

"I don't want to see your faces for the next seven days." There was pindrop silence. Nobody understood what Mr. Bindra was talking about.

"What sir?"

"I don't want to see your faces for the next seven days." Mr. Bindra repeated.

"Why sir?"

"Because I know you have worked for the last few months like mad, leaving your family and personal interests behind. I am granting all of you seven days official paid leave. Just go back homes and enjoy with your family. Forget the factory for the next seven days. This is a special gift to you from the management." Mr. Bindra told us with a rare smile on his face.

Everybody was stunned.

"Thank you sir." Everybody said in chorus.

"Mr. Roy (our Personnel manager) has arranged a bus for you to go back home right now. Is that clear?"

"Clear sir." Mr. Bindra left the conference hall and the group of officers went home.

54

LEARNING VALIDATION

It was a Sunday morning; we were not in our homes but were assembled in the Ranbaxy's guest house meeting room in the city.

Mr. Prafulla Seth, our Executive Vice-President (manufacturing) was in the city and he had called an urgent meeting. Most of the key people of the plant were present.

Mr. Seth started addressing the meeting. The meeting actually lasted for not more than 15 minutes, but yet the Sunday was spoilt.

"Good morning gentlemen. I have called a meeting at very short notice and I am glad to see you all here. Please excuse me for spoiling your Sunday morning, but I definitely will not take too much of your time, because I have to rush to the airport to catch my flight to Delhi."

Mr. Seth made a brief introduction to the meeting and continued further,

"You all know that we have already showed sufficient progress in the construction of our Plant – C for Cephalosporins, the facility validation and equipment validation of this plant is going to be very important and critical since we are going for MCA approval for this facility."

"I feel a separate validation team is required to be created to take this responsibility. I will send a bunch of books on validation and some files and write-ups which I received from our UK consultants. The team should study the whole thing, understand and implement them. I think Mr. Bindra and Mr. Agarwal will take the necessary steps in this regard. What do you say Mr. Bindra?"

"Yes sir. We will." Mr. Bindra assured Mr. Seth.

The meeting got over and all of us dispersed to enjoy the Sunday. The next day while I was eating hot samosa in the canteen with Dr. Kalidas, we received a message from our office peon which said that Mr. Bindra wants both of us in his office. (Those were the "non-mobile" days.)

"Good morning Sir," we greeted Mr. Bindra.

While entering his room, we saw Mr. Agarwal also joining us simultaneously.

"Sit down gentlemen."

We occupied the seats in front of Mr. Bindra. His table was crowded with some books and files, an unusual scene.

"Dr. Potdar, Mr. Seth has sent these books and some other reading materials on validation."

"Yes sir."

"You and Kalidas take all this to your office, read and analyse. We have to carry out the facility and equipments validation of the new plant." Bindra said.

"No problem sir, we will read and implement it under your guidance." Dr. Kalidas spoke while simultaneously looking at the pile of books on Dr. Bindra's table.

"What? Under my guidance? No, no, I don't know much about this validation and all. It is all you both have to study, understand and implement. I can only provide you anything you need. That's all. Everything you have to manage. May be Mr. Agarwal can provide you some help but definitely not me." Mr. Bindra cleared his stand.

Kalidas and I looked at each other while Mr. Agarwal was looking at both of us.

"Okay. Is that clear doctor?"

"Yes sir." I replied.

We collected the books and other materials and left his office and Mr. Bindra's table became clear as usual.

I still remember that day because it was the beginning of the study of pharmaceutical validation for me as well as Kalidas.

The entire following month we spent a lot of time reading and understanding what exactly validation means. We used to sit up late, have tea, discuss and try to find a path to proceed through the vast jungle of validation.

Believe me, till that day I was really not aware of what validation is all about but within a month's time we had a fair grasp of the subject.

The first document we made after this was a plan of activities on the expected scope of validation work in the plant. This rough scribbling finally took the shape of the "Validation Master File" which, when we showed Mr. Agarwal and Mr. Bindra, was highly appreciated and motivated us further by telling us that, Mr. Bindra will have a regular weekly meeting on the progress of validation work along with Mr. Agarwal and both of us.

Then gradually other people joined us as team members like Ramesh, Sunil, Devendra Joshi; who was our Engineering Manager and others. This small beginning made by us ultimately resulted into the successful completion of the validation work and approval by the MCA also.

This was the status of validation twenty three years back, but now? Even the most junior pharmacist in a pharma plant knows what validation is. What a wonderful transformation!

55

VIDEO TAPING OF VALIDATION

When we were going through the MCA audit preparation, in Ranbaxy one of the main activities was facility and equipment validation.

Mr. Bindra had distributed the work amongst selected senior executives and managers. The validation activity was given to Dr. Kalidas Sinha and me. Dr Kalidas Sinha was a chemical engineer with B.tech, M.tech and Ph.D (Tech) in chemical engineering from I.I.T Kharagpur. He was a very intelligent, hard-working and highly compatible person. Our team was really good, because I was familiar with pharma aspects, being a pharmacist by education, and Kalidas was thorough with engineering. He was also strong in mathematical and statistical aspects; and above all we were highly compatible with each other. We knew each other's strengths and weaknesses and we were trying to use our strengths in a synergistic manner. Mr. Bindra was also happy with our work.

We started validating the facilities and utilities i.e. mainly HVAC system and other systems too.

During these validation activities, Ramesh was also involved. He was taking care of the validation documentation. Lots of validation data was pouring in and it was necessary that the data be organised and compiled properly. This was a very tough job but Ramesh was managing this well along with his routine job of production management of his plant.

Lot of organised data was now in place, number of files were rapidly increasing. Each AHU validation was a file in itself and the number of AHUs were also very high. If I remember correctly the Cephalosporin block has nothing less than thirty AHUs. (Maybe little less or more)

Mr. Bindra gave us a suggestion: video tape the HVAC validation activities, and if possible even the equipment validation activities too. We started with video-taping the HVAC validation. We hired a video grapher and taped practically all HVAC activities along with the date and time simultaneously recorded. This video-tapes showed when a particular activity was carried out and who were involved in carrying out those activities.

We showed this to Mr. Bindra, Mr. Agarwal and all the other people involved in the validation activity.

This gave us two main advantages. One: it became a visual record of the validation activities carried out and two: since we were to show this to the auditors, all the people who worked on the project got highly motivated, because their involvement will be appreciated and this was really a great boost for the entire team.

When the validation task was over for the occasion i.e. whatever we had planned to complete before the MCA audit, we made an index of files which was quite a big number, but it was organised in such a way that retrieval of any system was very easy.

Similarly we made an index of video clippings in chronological fashion listing what activity was carried out on which day. Using this index it would be easy to retrieve the video of any specific activity that the auditor may want to see.

Since every activity was not videotaped, we marked in the files (paper documents) which activities were videotaped and which were not. So by studying the paper documents you would know which activities could be watched on a television screen.

The preparation was perfect. Just a day before the audit we arranged all the files in the conference room. Systematically the video tapes were kept with Mr. Bindra in his office.

On the second day of the audit, the inspector fixed the time of 3 o' clock for discussing the validation activities. I was to give the presentation on the validation activities to the auditors.

Everyone concerned with the activity was present in the conference room. Mr. Bindra asked me to present the validation activities related to the Cephalosporin plant.

I welcomed everybody and started my presentation. I gave one single A4 page executive summary of what I was going to present. I also gave two index papers one of validation files and the other of the video clippings.

I presented in brief the activities which were performed and the people who participated in the activities and showed the index wise organised files to the auditors, and also told them that if they want to see any specific thing from this we can show them along with the relevant documents.

"What is the video list Dr. Potdar?" One of the inspectors asked me.

"Sir amongst the activities related primarily to HVAC and facility, some of these we have videotaped and they are chronologically edited. Of course every activity is not video recorded but those which we thought were critical we have recorded and that is given in the list of video recordings, which is with you."

"Was there any specific reason for this?"

"Yes we thought videotaping is the most genuine record of the actual activity carried out. You actually see the people working on the task, whom you have met over the last two days. Of course we have all the documents in paper form as well, which is mandatory, but we thought of doing something not really mandatory but useful and genuine." I explained.

"Good. Thank you Dr. Potdar. Can we see some of the video shoots?"

"Yes of course."

We showed them a part of the video shoot, depending on what they wanted to see. They were really very happy to see that our plan was successful. They realised that Ranbaxy stands for genuine work. It goes without saying that we got the MCA approval in the first run itself.

56

ON THE BANK OF THE RIVER KSHIPRA

River Kshipra which flows through Indore and Ujjain and goes further is considered a holy river, but this holy river once put us in a serious problem. The problem definitely was not of the river in any way, it was of the people who used the water and banks of the river for their own purpose.

It was a cool winter morning in Indore, that day I was not in my car. I was travelling to our Ranbaxy plant in Mr. Agarwal's car with Dr. Willows. Mr. Agarwal and Dr. Willows were sitting in the back seat and I was in the front seat beside the driver. Dr. Willows was in the seat behind the driver.

The car was going smoothly, we crossed Lasudia and Manglia and we were on the Kshipra bridge. Suddenly Dr. Willows shouted, "Mr. Agarwal, please stop the car."

The driver heard this and took the car to one side of the bridge and stopped.

"What is the problem Dr. Willows? Do you want anything?" Mr. Agarwal asked.

"No I don't want anything, but I see something on the right side of the river bank."

"What?"

"Look, look at that side." Dr. Willows said, pointing to the right hand side of the bank where there were some yellow clothes kept for drying.

"Dr. Potdar, do you see those clothes there, the yellow ones?"

"Yes I see them there."

"Don't they look like Ranbaxy's yellow uniforms?"

Now I looked very carefully at them. They were definitely the Ranbaxy uniforms, drying on the river bank. I was about to say something but Mr. Agarwal interrupted and said, "No, no, no they are definitely not our company uniforms. We give our company uniforms to a laundry in Dewas."

"That may be the case but the laundry man may be washing them in the river water and drying them on the river bank."

"Can't be" Mr. Agarwal was trying to insist that they were not our uniforms but Dr. Willows was quite firm.

"Dr. Potdar, can you please go there and check?" Dr. Willows asked me.

I did not have any choice but to go.

"Okay I will go and check." I said.

I crossed the bridge and went to the river bank where the clothes were kept for drying on the rocks. I checked and saw that they were our uniforms. Then I came back.

"Well, what was that?" Dr. Willows asked.

"They were our uniforms. I will call the laundry man today to the factory and talk to him about this." I said.

We sat in the car. The car moved to the factory. We straight away went to Mr. Agarwals cabin. His secretary ordered some tea and biscuits for us.

"Dr. Potdar, remember one thing, it is not enough to appoint a laundry but you must go and see his laundering facility. Is it not?" Dr. Willows told me.

"Yes sir." I agreed.

"Having a SOP is not enough; the words have meaning only if their spirit is understood." Willows was talking the basic philosophy.

"Mr. Agarwal, I suggest that we get an inhouse laundry service for our uniform washing, alternatively you find a really good industrial launderer for our purpose, who has a really good facility and capacity to meet our laundering requirements."

"You are right Dr. Willows. I will make an immediate proposal for in-house laundry facility for us." Mr. Agarwal agreed.

Shortly we had our own facility for washing the uniforms.

57

FUN OF WORKING ON PROJECTS

On May 16th, 1994 I joined Wockhardt as General Manager (Production) to look after their new project at Daman, in Silver Industrial Estate.

Wockhardt had a plot of land in Silver Industrial Estate. When I joined it was just a barren piece of land, where the new factory was to be constructed, and I was supposed to look after this project, and run the factory after construction.

This was the first experience in my life: that of managing a project. I had worked in many companies as Production Manager, Plant Manager, etc. But I never handled a new factory project myself. Of course I had some experience about this when we had constructed Ranbaxy's third plant at Dewas, but at that time I was not heading the project myself. Even though I was associated with it, it was handled by my friend, Mr. Modi.

I joined the site in peak summer and the rainy season was to start just after 2-3 weeks. I was told that the rain in Daman tends to very heavy.

I had one close associate with me by name Mr. Mohammad Raja, who used to be a production Manager in our Aurangabad factory and was transferred to Daman.

Only the two of us were senior persons and all other primarily some skilled workmen were transferred from our Aurangabad factory. They were about ten of them.

Life on the site was going to be tough particularly when the rains start. We arranged for a site office which was a thin shed that had two small tables, a few plastic chairs and a pedestal fan. There were no arrangements for tea or lunch, in fact there was nothing there. There was no canteen or hotel near the construction site, and even for a cup of tea we had to walk nearly a kilometre.

We had a worker couple with us by name Mr. and Mrs Bhosale. Initially there was very little work for all the workers. Only Raja and I had lots of work to do. We would start work and every day at about 10:00 A.M. we used to go for tea to a small hotel near-by and we used to have our lunch there itself. It was hectic but we were managing.

Then one day Mr. Bhosale came to me and said, "Sir if you don't mind, I have a suggestion to make."

"Yes tell me." I said. Raja and I were sitting in our so called office.

"Sir it is very tiring for you and Raja sahib to go for tea every morning to that small tapri type hotel."

"I know." I said.

"Sir, my wife says if you make some arrangements for an electric heater and some utensils, she will make tea for all of us and we need not go to that small hotel all the way there."

"I think it is a good idea. What do you say Raja?" I asked.

"Yes sir, if Bhosale bhabhi can make the tea we can arrange for an electric heater and some untensils. "

"Meanwhile we will see if we can get some person to do this job during our project work."

"Thank you sir." Bhosale was really very happy.

I asked Mr. Bhosale to get the necessary utensils and electric heater from the market.

We started making tea in the office and slowly biscuits and toasts etc. also got added and a joint family type organisational structure got developed on the site. There was no formal organisational structure in the beginning of the project. It was me, the General Manager; Mr. Raja, the Production Manager; and all the other people were workers. But when we had our first sip of tea made my Mrs Bhosale, it was the beginning of a joyous project life which we enjoyed right up to the very end of the project.

We had some funny instances during these project days, I will narrate one or two of those. But what is important here is that after that we never felt project work to be a burden, it was more of a wonderful and pleasant life that we led.

It was a rainy day in the month of July. I was to make some documents to be submitted to the factory inspector. Raja and I both were not fully acquainted with what had to be submitted. I had one friend by name Mr. B. C. Shekar who was the factory Manager of Medley Pharmaceuticals Limited. We had the complete postal address of that place but had never been there. I wanted to see him and get some help for preparing the document.

"Raja, get ready, we have to go see Mr. Shekar at Medley Labs." I told Raja.

"Okay Sir, give me five minutes. I will be ready by then and we can leave."

"Okay."

Raja and I got ready and we started off in my car. It was raining heavily. We were going to the place given in the address.

We reached a place and we thought it would be better to check the address with some local person so that we may not miss the road. I stopped the car and started looking for someone to ask, and guide us. Raja opened the window on his side.

"Hello." He called to a passer-by, "Can you tell us how to reach Medley Pharma?" Raja asked. "Sir, go straight. On your right you will see a lake, take the turn to your left and from there you will be able to see the factory."

We were very happy that we were on the right path. We drove further on the road. Because of the heavy rain there was hardly anybody on the road. After a while we saw a small lake on our right side and a small road on the left. I stopped the car. "Raja I think this is the road on the left side, but I have a doubt because the road is small and you don't see anything on that road. Hope the man has told us correctly." I expressed my doubt.

"No Sir the road must be correct. He said take a left turn from the small lake and I don't see any other road on the left side. I think we can proceed down this road and see." Raja seemed quite confident. I turned the car to the left side of the small road. The road was small and on both sides of the road there was literally nothing. We continued to drive further till we reached a dead end and there was no way left to go. Rain was still pouring down. We were on the wrong track. We stopped.

Raja got down with his umbrella and started looking for someone to help us. But nobody was there. The road was so small and slippery that reversing the car was also difficult but we had no option.

"Raja, you stand on the road and guide me while I reverse the car." I said.

"Okay Sir."

I used all my skill and caution to reverse the car and finally came back to the point where we took the left turn. At that point we saw a local person. Raja quickly came out of the car and caught hold of that person. Both of them were close to the car on the driver's side, I rolled down my window glass.

"Hello we want to go to Medley" I started. The man stopped and asked me, "Saab Medley is still further. Why did you go on this small road?"

"We were told to take the left turn from this small lake."

"That is correct, but then why did you turn here? The lake is still further, about half a kilometre from here."

'What? Then what is this?" I pointed with my finger to the small water pool behind him.

"Oho…" he laughed and said, "Sir this is not a lake, this is only the accumulated rain water in the field, since it's been pouring really heavily for the last two days. This is not that lake, you please go further down the road and half a kilometre later you will see the lake and then you can take the left turn there, you will then reach Medley Pharma."

"Oh my god! Thank you very much gentleman." I heartily thanked the man.

We misunderstood the accumulated rain water in the fields as the lake to which the first person was referring and hence we had taken the left turn there. We went half a kilometre further down and found the real lake and the Medley factory to its left.

By now we had become familiar with the heavy rain of Daman. The site was full of mud and it was extremely difficult to walk on the site. We did not have any idea about the rainy season of Daman, so we had not taken any precautions to protect the site.

Raja and I had decided to purchase gum boots, because without gum boots it was just not possible to walk on the site. I asked Raja to purchase two pairs of gum boots for the both of us first and then we would make arrangements for the others.

Next day we reached our office site. Luckily the site office was on the side of the main road of the Silver Industries Estate, so there was no slush, as the main road was quite hard and good.

Raja showed me the gumboots. These gumboots were the low leg protection and not really the full leg protection type of gumboots.

"Raja I don't think these will work, I think we should get the full leg protection boots."

"No sir, the mud will not be so much. These will be sufficient."

"You have to try."

"Yes sir. I will change and go to the building site and see."

"Okay, shall we go together?" I asked.

"No, no Sir let me go first and see if the boots are fine."

"Be careful."

Raja wore the ankle sized gumboots, took an umbrella and left the office. I was looking at him while he was walking toward the main building that was being constructed. Suddenly I heard a scream from Raja.

"What happened Raja?" I asked in a worried tone.

"Sir, not only my shoe but half my leg is in the mud. I don't think this shoe will work."

'Come back Raja, come back."

"Sir it is difficult to walk."

"Wait Raja I am coming."

"Sir, you don't go, we will go and help Raja sir." Two site workers told me and went to rescue Raja.

Somehow the two workers managed to get Raja to the office. The lower part of his trouser was completely soiled by the mud. Somebody fetched a bucket of water to wash his feet and pants.

When the mud was washed Raja realised that his right shoe was missing.

"Sir, probably my right shoe got stuck in the mud itself and I didn't even realise that I was coming back with just one shoe." Raja explained.

"Leave it Raja, leave it." I said.

Funny incidents like this will occur at the construction site and one should just enjoy and learn from them.

58

SKY IS THE LIMIT
(Mr. JOSEPH'S CASE)

Work at Wockhardt Daman factory project was coming to a close and we were planning to start production. We had three formulations there to start with, tablets, capsules and liquid injectables.

The project which started with only two Managers and about ten workmen had now become quite a big group of production, quality control, engineering, warehouse i.e. more or less a full-fledged manufacturing unit.

We had a small administrative office, but we did not have any secretarial assistance, not even a typist. We used to get all our typing work done from a small typing shop from the town. Every day I used to collect the typing work and while going back home, I used to give the work to a typing shop owner, explain it to him and he used to get it done by the evening and would give it to me in the morning when I used to come to the factory.

Slowly the work increased and we started looking for a good typist for our factory on a temporary basis to start with.

In that typing shop there was a young South Indian boy, he may not have been even twenty. He was very smart, I used to explain the work to him and he used to do it with practically no mistakes at all.

Secondly he never used to delay the work. He used to keep the material ready at whatever time he had said it would be ready and sometimes he would even deliver the typed material to the factory.

One day he came to the factory with the typed work in the afternoon at about 3 PM. Our Personnel Head Mr. Guha had come from Mumbai since we had some interviews for the factory employment.

Mr. Joseph, that south Indian typist boy entered my room.

"Sir, your work." Joseph said.

"Thanks Joseph, good, please wait and see Mr. Raja on the first floor, and meet me before you go back."

"Okay Sir." Joseph said and left my room.

"What is this Doctor?" Mr. Guha asked me looking at the typed work.

"Sir presently we do not have a typist, as I told you, so we get it done from a small typing shop in the city. This fellow Joseph works there." I explained.

"Oh, I see. He is employed there by the shop owner is it?"

"Yes Sir."

"Is he a graduate?"

"I don't know sir, but his English is good and so is his typing."

"If he was a graduate we can consider him for the job as your secretary. Can you call him down?"

"Why not? I think it will be a very good idea." I contacted Raja on the intercom and asked him to send Joseph down.

"Yes sir, you called me?"

"Yes Joseph, have a seat."

"It is okay Sir." Joseph was a little hesitant to sit in front of us.

"Sit down, sit down Joe." Mr. Guha said.

Joseph sat down with a little hesitation.

"Tell me Joseph, how long have you been here in Daman?" Mr. Guha asked him.

Joseph did not understand why this gentleman was asking this question to him suddenly and without any reference to context.

"Joseph Mr. Guha is our Personnel Head. He has come to our factory to make some recruitments." I introduced Mr. Guha to Joseph.

Now Joseph suddenly became cautious. "For the last one year sir," he answered.

"What is you educational qualifications?"

"Sir I have passed my twelfth standard and completed a diploma in typing and Pitman's shorthand from Kerala."

"What is your speed?"

"Forty and hundred sir, I am really good at English typing."

"What are you doing other than your job presently?"

"Sir I am doing B.A. externally from IGNOU. I have already completed my first year and am currently pursuing my second year of a three year course." Joseph gave his educational and professional background.

"How much salary do you get at the present job?"

"Fifteen hundred a month sir."

"Good, okay see you Joe." Mr. Guha said as he concluded the interview.

"Joseph finish your work with Raja and then come and see me before leaving the factory." I told him.

"Yes sir, thank you sir." Joseph said as he left the room.

"Guha saab the boy is really good, hard-working and sincere." I told Mr. Guha.

"Yes I can see that, but the only problem is he is not a graduate and you know our company policy is that we must have a minimum graduate person for this job."

"I know but can we not make an exception to the rule? I can tell you this boy will be a graduate within the next eighteen months, plus he has a diploma in shorthand and typing also."

"Hmmmm… I know. Okay don't tell him anything right now. Tomorrow I will be back in Mumbai in the head office and I will discuss this with the MD, I think he will agree."

"Please sir, do that."

"I will." said Mr. Guha.

A week passed and I received a letter from Mr. Guha saying that the Head Office Management had agreed as an exceptional case to appoint Joseph on a temporary basis till he completes his graduation and then he will be absorbed as a regular employee.

I was really very happy. I thanked Mr. Guha. Joseph joined our Daman factory as my Secretarial Assistant. He demonstrated all his good qualities not only as a secretary but also as a person. He completed his BA in sociology and economics. He became a permanent staff of the factory.

I left Wockhardt after that and joined Intas Pharmaceutical in Ahmedabad. My brother was in Daman working for Medley Pharmaceuticals.

Once when I came to Daman to see my brother and we were in the market place and suddenly I heard someone calling out to me.

"Sir, sir, Potdar sir."

I turned around and saw that it was Joseph calling me.

"Hi Joseph. How are you man?"

"I am good sir, how are you and where are you now sir?"

"I am fine and I am right now working for Intas in Ahmedabad."

"That is nice sir."

"What are you doing these days Joe?"

"Sir I completed my MA in public administration and now working as an administrative officer in an engineering company here."

"Good, very good. Keep it up Joe."

"Thank you sir, it is all because of you. You gave me a chance to work with you. I learnt a lot of things while working with you sir."

"I only gave you the chance to work, all the rest was your efforts, hard work and sincerity."

"Thank you."

"Okay, see you."

"Thanks again." Joe said as he shook my hand and then left.

I know Joseph was an ordinary twelfth standard passed boy, but with all his good qualities he would have come up and no one could have stopped his progress.

59

USING MUSCLE POWER

This is a story of a company where I was working as a Location Head. The new factory was ready and I was to get the manufacturing license from the F.D.A. The plant was ready in all respects i.e., the building and equipment was ready, the lab equipment was in place, people employed, everything was ready. I had submitted the application with all required documents completed and double checked. Every necessary document was in place.

I met the concerned officer to request him for the inspection. He promised me that he would come within five to seven days and get my factory inspected and if found to be okay then he would issue a manufacturing license immediately.

First of all he delayed the factory inspection for more than three weeks and every time I met him he would give me some excuse and give me another date. Finally after nearly three weeks he came to the factory, inspected the factory, made his remarks and told me that everything seems okay. I will send my report to the Drug Controller who is supposed to issue the manufacturing license.

I was happy. I also did "All other things" which I was generally "supposed to do" as per the inspecting officer's suggestion. In fact he told that within three to four days I would receive the license. I thanked him.

I waited for one week, and there was no response from his office. I called him and his assistant too, but they did not give me any satisfactory reply. Finally I decided to meet the Drug Controller. I went to his office.

"Good morning Sir." I greeted the Drug Controller.

"Good morning Dr. Potdar." He reciprocated.

"Sir your officer inspected our factory for the purpose of getting a manufacturing license purpose. Now it has been more than two weeks. I have not received any information from him. The management is after me to start production. I need your help in this matter sir. In fact I have done "everything" which your officer told me. I don't know why he is taking so much time to give the license." I explained my situation.

"Okay let me check with him. He is not there today. Give me some time and I will get back to you." The D.C. told me.

"When should I contact you sir?"

"Don't worry I will call you back."

"When can I expect your call sir?" I was insisting.

"How can I say that Dr. Potdar? We have so many jobs to do, I don't have only your job at hand." The D.C was getting a little angry.

"I know sir. I know you have a lot of work, but I am facing a serious problem because of this delay. If you expect me to do "something more" please tell me. I am prepared to do that." I told him.

"What do you mean? I told you I will do it at the appropriate time. Please allow me to attend to my other duties and when I finish I will call you." The D.C indirectly suggested me to leave his office.

I waited for another one week and then called the D.C on the phone and asked him the status of my license. He replied that he has not yet received the inspection report from the officer and until he receives it, he cannot do anything and I just have to wait.

I was really frustrated. In that frustration I called my Managing Director in Mumbai and very briefly narrated the story to him. He listened quietly and gave me the name and number of a person and asked me to contact him and he would give me an appropriate direction to follow.

That very day I went to that man's office. He had a plastic materials factory, a well-known brand of plastic chairs, etc. was being manufactured in his factory. Secondly he was also the M.L.A of the ruling party.

I entered his office and gave my visiting card to the receptionist and told her that I wanted to meet the "Bade Saab."

"Please wait sir." The receptionist told me very decently.

"Thank you." I said.

I waited there for half an hour more and then I started to get uneasy.

"How much longer will it take madam?" I asked the receptionist

"Normally he meets visitors immediately. Let me just check if he is busy with some other things."

"Yes please do that."

She checked with his secretary. The secretary came out of the cabin.

"Sir, are you Dr. Potdar?" the secretary asked me.

"Yes." I said.

"Saab has asked you to come in."

"Thank you." I entered the boss' cabin.

The cabin was well decorated, there was a big table with a clean glass top, mild light in the room and a middle aged person, looking very decent and sober sitting in the boss' chair.

"Good morning sir." I greeted the bade saab.

"Good morning doctor, please sit down, I am sorry, you had to wait. Generally I don't like people being kept waiting. Tell me what can I do for you?"

Believe me I never expected such a decent and sober welcome by a factory owner cum an M.L.A of the ruling party of the state.

"Thank you so much sir for giving me your valuable time." I was being a little more formal.

'No need to be so formal doctor. Tell me, what can I do for you?"

"Sir I am the head of the factory and I am waiting for the manufacturing license from the F.D.A. All formalities have been completed, I mean all the documents have been submitted, the officer had inspected our factory, I also did "what other things he expected me to do." He had a typical smile on his face but I still have not received the license. Our M.D is your personal friend, he advised me to take your help in this regard." I briefly narrated to the bade saab.

"Tell me who is supposed to give you the license?"

"The Drug Controller sir."

"Do you have his name and number with you?"

"Yes sir." I gave him the name and the number. He asked his secretary to connect him to the D.C.

"Sir D.C on the line" the secretary handed the receiver to him.

"Good morning sir. I have Dr. Potdar here of XXX company sitting in front of me. I understand his manufacturing license is pending for your signature in your office. Dr. Potdar will see you at four in the evening. You hand over the duly signed license into his hands. Thanks."

The bade saab put the receiver down. "You may go now Dr. Potdar and collect your license at four in the evening and just call me after receiving it." He said.

"Sir, did he say he will give it?" I asked with little hesitation.

"Who D.C? Why should I ask him, if he is going to give it? No, no no need. You will get it. " he said with complete confidence and a pleasing smile on his face.

I finished the last sip of coffee from the cup and left his office.

I went back to the factory and had my lunch and left the office at about 4 P.M to see the D.C at his office.

The DC's office had a big entrance in the corridor. I parked my car and started walking in the corridor to reach the D.C's office.

I saw someone at the other end of the corridor with some paper in their hand. I walked further, the man started approaching me. Now I could see his face clearly, it was the D.C.

"Good evening sir." I greeted him.

"Good evening Dr. Potdar. See these are your three manufacturing licenses." He handed over the license to me.

"Thanks." I said.

"You should have told me. Why did you go to bade saab?" the D.C asked me.

"I approached you twice, you know I am under pressure from the management to start production sir, understand my situation." I replied.

"Okay, okay. Please call bade saab and tell him that you received the manufacturing license. In future if you have any problem, come straight to me. Don't go anywhere else. After all we are friends yaar. And don't forget to tell bade saab without fail." He repeatedly insisted to me.

I assured him that I would tell bade saab and left the office.

I drove straight to the Bade ssab's office and showed him the license and thanked him for his help. 'If you ever get stuck up somewhere do not hesitate to come to me." He told me, as I was leaving the office.

Sometimes it is essential to take help from such people but never make it a practice.

60

INTERVIEW IN CADILA PHARMA

In pharma companies or for that matter any company you meet different types of people and face different situations.

I still remember my interview day with Cadila Pharma. I was called for the interview at 11:00 AM in the morning. I reached at about ten forty and told the receptionist that I have an interview with Dr. Rajeev Modi at 11:00 AM. She asked me to wait in the reception, gave me a glass of water and asked if I would like a cup of tea.

"No thanks" I said and sat on the sofa in the reception hall looking at some magazines kept on the table there. I was looking at my wrist watch uneasily and the receptionist also kept occasionally glancing at me and giving me a smile, probably meaning that Dr. Rajeev is busy and you have to wait for some more time. Dr. Rajeev was the Managing Director of the company.

It was nearly half past twelve, nearly two hours had passed since I arrived and still I was not called in. I started to get uncomfortable. The receptionist observed my discomfort. I knew the receptionist because she worked in Cadila Labs Limited where I was the Production controller.

At about 1:00 PM she told me that she had arranged for my lunch in the management canteen and I should have my lunch since it was already lunch time and if Dr. Rajeev calls me, she would tell him that

I had gone for lunch and that I would meet him immediately after lunch.

But I declined her request and asked if I could see Dr. Rajeev's secretary in his office.

She checked with Dr. Rajeev's secretary.

"Dr. Potdar you may go to the fourth floor and see Dr. Rajeev's secretary. She has called you."

"Thanks" I said and went to Dr. Rajeev's office to see his secretary.

"Hello Dr. Potdar, we are meeting after a long time, how are you? Please sit down." Dr. Rajeev's secretary greeted me with a warm smile.

"Yes really, it has been a long time. How are you? How is it going?"

"Good, as it should be." She gave a guarded reply.

'see I was waiting downstairs from 11:00 in the morning, the boss gave me an appointment at eleven sharp and now it is half past one."

"I know, you see expectedly today some foreign delegates had come and Dr. Rajeev is busy with them but he knows about your appointment. In fact he even told me about your meeting."

"See, I want to go out and come in the evening, can you please postpone my appointment to say four thirty or so in the evening?" I asked.

"I think it is possible. So should I keep it at four thirty?"

"Yes, thank you very much."

"It is alright doctor."

"Okay see you at four thirty." I said and left the office.

I came down and straight away I went home to have lunch. There I narrated the entire story to my wife. I told her that I would relax for some time but had to leave at four sharp since I had to be back in the office by four thirty to see Dr. Rajeev.

I reached the office again at about four twenty or so. I requested the receptionist to convey to Dr. Rajeev's secretary that I had come, since she has given me an appointment at four thirty with Dr. Rajeev.

"But Dr. Potdar, Dr. Rajeev has still not come back from the lunch with the foreign delegates. Of course he may be coming back at any moment. You may sit here or if you prefer you may sit in his office with his secretary."

"No I will stay at the reception itself."

"As you wish."

"Thanks."

You will not believe Dr. Rajeev came back with his guests at about five thirty, I was still waiting and continued to wait in the reception till about eight thirty at night, totally tired and very frustrated.

At about nine in the night I was called up. I was tired of sitting for such a long time and so I decided to take the stairs. I reached the fourth floor and to my surprise I saw Dr. Rajeev had already closed the door to his office and was standing outside his office with a bunch of papers in his hand.

"Good morning, I mean good evening sir." I fumbled with my greetings.

"Nothing wrong in saying good morning, because I had called you in the morning only." Dr. Rajeev joked and I just smiled and looked at him.

"Sir I was supposed to have an interview."

"What interview?"

"The interview that you had called me for sir."

"I know but I know you for so long when you were working in Cadila Labs with me."

"Yes sir."

"So, do one thing, tomorrow meet Mr. Sabarwal in his office in the morning and discuss your pay packet with him. He knows all about you and the job which you are here for. Okay?"

"Yes sir."

"Good, now good night doctor, and tell him that he must clear your papers tomorrow itself and send them to me for my signature before five in the evening."

"Yes sir."

"And join the job as soon as you can as there is a lot of work waiting for you here."

"Okay sir thank you."

"Okay and good night again."

I left the office within five minutes.

The interview had lasted not more than ten minutes for which I had waited almost ten hours.

61

First Day in Cadila Pharma

My interview for the position of General Manager (Mfg. Technologies.) was a great event as I have described earlier.

I joined the company when Cadila's new pharma plant was being constructed at Dholka about fifty kilometres from Ahmedabad city. My collegemate, just 3 years junior to me in B. Pharm. Mr. S.G. Hardikar was also working with the same company as General Manager (Production).

I was supposed to be reporting to Mr. Sri Ram Khanna who was Vice-President (projects) for a new plant, and I was responsible for facility, equipment and process validation of the new plant, which was expected to be ready in another 8-10 months' time.

I reported for duty at sharp eight in the morning and met Mr. Sri Ram Khanna, my boss. We were in our Head Office in Ahmedabad.

Mr. S.R. Khanna very briefly informed me about the project. I met the project engineer Mr. Lalitbhai Champaneria, who was earlier working with me in Cadila Laboratories Ltd, when I was the Production Controller of the company. We spent quite some time together talking about the new project of Dholka.

At about 1:00 P.M Mr. S.R. Khannna called me. "Potdar we are going to Dholka site." He just told me.

"Okay sir."

"Come on we are getting late."

"Yes." I said as I picked up my briefcase and followed him. That day I had not brought my car and so we travelled in Mr. Khanna's car. It took about an hour to reach the site. The facility was in an advanced stage of construction.

We entered the site office. There were two engineers and some other people in the office. It was about 2:00 P.M. and I was feeling very hungry. I had not had any breakfast also since I had left my home very early in the morning.

Since it was my first day in the new office, I was not even aware that there was a canteen facility or any other thing. My boss never showed any concern for the newly joined employee. He was fully aware that it was well past lunch time and courtesy demanded that he at least ask me about having some food. But that type of courtesy was totally missing in this new boss.

He took me around the site. We moved around the site for about an hour and came back to the site office at about 3:00 P.M. or so.

Finally I lost my patience and asked him, "Sir are we not going to have lunch?"

"We will but the work is more important." He replied.

"Do you have some eating facility on the site?" I asked.

He looked at me very strangely as if I had asked something very unusual question.

"I have also not had anything since morning."

"Then why don't we eat something and then continue with the work?" I also started responding to him in his own style.

Luckily at the same time a boy came up to Mr. Khanna and asked, "Sir will you have some lunch? The Manager has asked me to check with you."

"Yes both of us, him and myself are going to have lunch." I told that boy.

Mr. Khanna looked at me somewhat annoyed.

"Bring something here in the office." Mr. Khanna told the boy. The boy ran to the site canteen to get food for us.

"Some people are more concerned about eating than work." I heard Mr. Khanna's words but I decided to ignore that.

We had our lunch and once again Mr. Khanna got immersed with his work. I got hold of a site engineer and went for a stroll around the site. I came back at about six in the evening and found that Mr. Khanna was still busy with the work in the office.

I was little worried as I did not have a mobile phone with me at that time since I had just shifted to Ahmedabad a few days back. I did not have a fixed landline phone either. In fact there was no way that I could have communicated to my wife that I was held up at the construction site and may come only late in the night. Remember it was my very first day in the new company. Even if I became really late she had no way to contact anyone to find out about my whereabouts. Meanwhile I asked Mr. Khanna, "Sir when will we be going back?"

"After the work is over." He replied curtly.

There was no point in asking him when the work would get over and so I kept quiet.

Finally we left the site at about twelve in the night and it was 1 A.M. by the time I reached home and saw that my wife was literally in tears.

This was my first day in Cadila Pharmaceuticals Ltd.

I remember what my Personnel Manager and also my friend had told me once, that the new employee will decide on day one whether he will continue with an organisation or not.

What a true statement.

62

MEETING AT 6.00 A.M.

Dr. Rajeev Modi of Cadila was a young dynamic man and a total workaholic. He was also highly educated and intelligent person. He obtained his B. tech in chemical engineering from IIT and thereafter his M.S and Ph. D in biochemical engineering from U.S.A.

Even if he worked ten to fourteen hours a day he would not seem tired. Trying to matching his stamina and dedication for work was next to impossible for anyone in the company at that time.

Once we had a meeting in the head office on a Saturday evening. The meeting started at about four and about five thirty Dr. Rajeev decide to close the meeting and continue at another time since he had another important engagement.

"So gentlemen we will close the meeting for now and continue tomorrow at 6:00 A.M." Dr. Rajeev said.

"Yes sir, we will leave the factory a little early and reach here before six in the evening." one of my colleagues said.

"What?" Dr. Rajeev was terribly annoyed.

Everyone was shocked.

"Is the factory running tomorrow?"

"No sir."

"Then what do you mean by you will leave the factory a little early and reach here by six?"

Everyone realised that the colleague who said that had assumed two things; first, that tomorrow meant the next working day, whereas Dr. Rajeev meant tomorrow as the next day itself i.e. Sunday and second my friend thought that when Dr. Rajeev said 6 AM he actually meant 6 P.M and it was just a slip of the tongue. But it was not a slip of the tongue at all. You could not expect such things from Dr. Rajeev.

The meeting was held the next day itself i.e. on Sunday and at six in the morning and not in the evening.

It was very hectic but also fun working for Cadila Pharma.

63

RAGHUVIR MANGALURKAR – THE GOAN CONNECTION

C.F.L Pharmaceuticals Pvt. Ltd. is a Goa based company of Menezes group.

C.F.L stands for Cosme Farma Laboratories. (A Portugese time company and Farma means Pharma) I was to go to attend an interview with this company in their Mumbai Head Office, for the position of Production Manager.

I had some time on my hands to prepare for the interview. Looking at the name of the company, I thought the company must be manufacturing cosmetics and pharmaceuticals, since its name contained both 'cosme' and 'farma'. I prepared myself for both aspects and went for the interview.

The interview was conducted by Mr. Menezes, the General Manager of the company and son of the owner. But he did not ask any questions on cosmetics. I was little surprised about it but I did not bother.

I got selected for the post and joined as Production Manager.

The company was in a small town of Ponda in Goa. I was provided a very big flat in the building called "Bhavani Sadan". This building was earlier owned by the Chief Minister of Goa, Mr. Dayanand Bandadkar.

I reached Ponda with my wife and my two kids. I had two days with me before I had to join the factory so I decided to help my wife get settled in the new house. Both of us arranged the entire house in two days. The only thing that could not be settled was the cooking gas. The gas agent had told me that if we submitted the papers related to the earlier gas connection we might get our connection within ten to fifteen days. So I arranged for a kerosene stove and some kerosene to make do with until our gas arrived. Both of us, my wife and I, were a little disturbed by the non-availability of the cooking gas. But we had no other choice but to manage with the kerosene stove.

I reported to the factory, my boss was Mr. Raghuvir Mangalurkar, who was the General Manager of Production and the Location Head. He had four production units under his control. Each unit had a Production Manager and all four of us were reporting to Mr. Raghuvir Mangalurkar.

I went to report to him on the first floor where his office was. Mr. Mangalurkar was a middle aged and mature executive. He had earlier worked with companies like Hoechst and Glaxo and had been trained in U.K by Shulton company whose 'Old-Spice' brand we were manufacturing in Goa in our group of companies.

Mr. Mangalurkar had a very warm and magnetic personality. He warmly welcomed me and asked me about whether I had settled in properly or not, whether the home was settled or not and also asked me about how my children are doing and about their schooling etc.

Then he called Mr. Mahendra Alve, who was Assistant Production Manager and was supposed to be reporting to me. He was a very young and sober pharmacist. I realised that he knew his job well.

Mr. Mangularkar introduced me to Mahendra and asked him to take me around the factory. Things were going smooth.

My wife got fed up with the kerosene stove and was always after me to get the cooking gas. I tried but the agent would always give me some reason or the other and I got really tired of that.

That day I came to the factory in a disturbed mood. Mr. Mangalurkar saw me and realised something is wrong. He called me to his office.

"Good morning sir." I said as I entered Mr. Mangalurkar's office.

"Come, come sit down." He said.

"Thank you sir."

"Manohar you don't seem to be in your normal mood today. Is there any problem?"

"Nothing specific."

"Then what? Something is there."

"Actually sir for the past two weeks we have been trying to get a cooking gas connection and somehow we have not been able to get it. I have submitted all my papers also. My wife is getting fed up using the kerosene stove." I explained to him.

"Oh, that is nothing."

"I know."

"How is everything in the plant? How is Mahendra?"

"Absolutely no problem. There is no problem with the factory working and Mahendra is a really good person."

"How old is your son?" he asked me.

"Just two and a half sir."

"Okay, so no problem about school this year."

"Yes sir."

"Good, don't worry you will get the gas. If you have any problem please feel free to come to and talk to me. Okay?"

"Okay sir. Thank you." I said and left his office.

The problem of the cooking gas was still in my mind. I used to go home for lunch every day at about twelve thirty and used to see the frustrated look on my wife's face because of the non-availability of the gas.

As usual I reached home that day for lunch and to my surprise I saw my wife with a very very bright and smiling face.

"Baba, Aai has made a sweet dish today for lunch." My son Sagar told me the moment I entered the house.

"My god! What for? What is the special occasion?"

"You arranged for a gas connection from your factory no? That man from your factory came over today and fixed the gas and left." My wife told me.

"I sent a gas connection from the factory? No, I don't know anything about that."

"What? But the man said he came from CFL factory to fix the gas." My wife said.

"I have to check." I said.

I had my lunch with the special sweet dish to celebrate the arrival of the gas and then went back to the factory. I staright away went to Mr. Mangalurkar's office.

"May I come in sir?"

"Yes, by all means."

"Sir, did you send somebody to my house with the cooking gas?" I asked.

"Did you get it?"

"Yes sir."

"Yes I sent it from my home, I had an extra gas cylinder with me. You are going to get your gas connection after three days. I called your agent and he promised me that." Mr. Mangalurkar told me.

I realised one important thing from Mr. Mangalurkar, that manager's duty is to see that his people are comfortable if you want them to concentrate on their work.

Once I talked to my boss Mr. Mangalurkar about my interview and asked him, "Sir when CFL is not manufacturing any cosmetics then why is the word 'cosme' there in the name of the company?"

Mr. Mangalurkar laughed from deep within his heart and said, "Manohar that word 'cosme' is not in any way related to cosmetics but it is the name of the founder of this company 'Cosme Mathias Menezes'." I joined in his laughter.

64

SIMPLE IPQC TECHNIQUES

CFL was a really small company but it has certain simple techniques developed for IPQC. I was told that these simple instruments were designed and got fabricated by Mr. Mangalurkar.

One of these instruments was for measuring viscosity of an intermediate liquid stage of making suspension. We were to measure the viscosity as an IPQC test and every time the sample had to be taken and sent to the Q.C lab and the manufacturing pharmacist had to wait before proceeding to the next step of manufacturing until he got the results back from the lab.

Mr. Mangalurkar designed a simple device. He took a hundred ml burette and attached in such a way in the liquid department that the liquid whose viscosity was to be measured would flow through it. The operator and the pharmacist would note down the time taken for 100 ml of that particular liquid to flow through the burette. He asked the Q.C person to collaborate the time limits in which the viscosity will be in acceptable limits. And the time limits were given to the manufacturing pharmacist and this really worked. Now the pharmacist did not have to wait for the viscosity results to proceed to the further steps in manufacturing.

A similar simple device was also designed by him for measuring tablet thickness of various tablet products during compression operations.

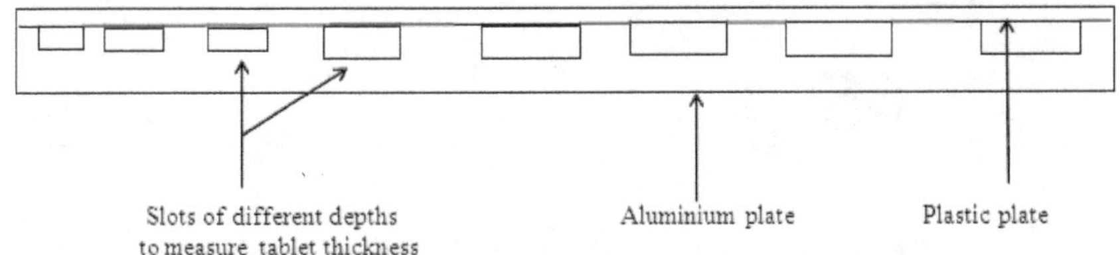

An aluminium plate was taken of about 20 × 20 × 0.5 cm dimension and different thickness slots cut out in that as shown in the diagram, and a transparent poly carbonate plate was fixed on its side. The slot represents the thickness of the tablets and the operator is required to just drop the tablet from one end and see if the tablet goes through the channel smoothly. In fact this represents the strip sealing channel, so that the operator need not actually check the thickness of the tablet using a vernier calipers.

I think the production pharmacist should develop such simple devices for machine operators which saves time. The pharmacist may however check the actual dimensions/ values and record it in the IPQC charts.

65

Matinee with Director

When I was working with CFL the factory was in Ponda, about 30 km from Panaji where we had our head office.

Every month we used to have our Production review meeting at HO. It used to start at about ten in the morning and get over in about two hours. Then we used to go back to the factory.

One such day Mr. Karnataki, our R and D Manager was with me for the meeting and for some reason the meeting concluded in an hour itself and we were free by eleven. We left the office to go back to the factory. On the way there was a cinema theatre. Mr. Karnataki saw a poster of a famous old English movie in the front of the cinema theatre. The movie was at eleven thirty and we decided to go.

"Manohar chal yaar this is a good movie. Let us go for it and then go to the factory." Karnataki said.

"No yaar this is very close to the Head Office. If the director sees us here we had it." I said.

But Karnataki made me agree and finally we got two tickets and went to see the movie.

I was a little uncomfortable at the thought of going for the movie while on duty. During the interval, we didn't go out but continued to sit inside the theatre itself.

"Karnataki see if anybody sees us here I am going to tell them that you forced me to come to the movie. " I said jokingly.

"Don't worry yaar nobody will see, everybody is busy in the office." Karnataki said.

Suddenly we heard a voice from behind us.

"Not everybody is busy in the office. I am here behind you."

We were shocked and surprised. We turned around and saw our director's son; Mr. Conrad Menezes sitting behind us.

"Oh my god! Conrad what are you doing here?" I asked.

"The same thing that you are doing." He said.

Conrad was studying in a pharmacy college in his final year of B. Pharamacy at that time and he used to come to the factory to learn the factory operations.

"Don't worry sir, I am not going to tell papa that you came to see the movie while on office duty provided you don't tell him that I bunked college and came here."

"No, of course not." We said.

We enjoyed the movie and after that Conrad went to college and we went back to the factory.

66

We Work only Half Day on Saturday

Personnel Managers are always brilliant guys.

I finished my interview with the Managing Director Mr. Nimish Bhai of Intas Pharmaceuticals Ltd. and had a meeting with Mr. Shaha, the Vice-President of Personnel.

First of all the compensation related issues were discussed and agreed upon. Then he talked about various aspects of factory working etc. which he thought would be useful to me as the Head of Production.

Meanwhile a person came in and served us tea and we continued our discussion. "Doctor Potdar, we work only half a day on Saturday." Mr. Shaha told me while talking about holidays and the leave patterns in the company.

"Oh that is good." I said.

The discussion was over. I left his office. I joined the company after about twenty days. After I joined the company I realised that the plant had Saturday as its weekly off and that meant the factory was working six days a week officially. I was wondering why Mr. Shaha told me that Saturday we work only for half a day. Then I realised that although Saturday was our weekly off, most Saturdays we spent our mornings in the factory.

What a good joke.

67

DO YOU HAVE AN SOP ON LAWN MOWING

When I was working in Intas Pharmaceuticals Ltd. as Vice-President (Technical) in the year 2000, we were scheduled for a TGA, Australia audit for our Ahmedabad plant.

The audit was for three days. On the morning of our second day when we were having coffee with our auditors one of the auditors, suddenly asked a funny question. (I thought it was funny but actually it was not.)

"Doctor Potdar, do you have an SOP on lawn mowing?" the auditor asked.

Everyone at the coffee table looked surprised. I looked at him for a moment with a puzzled expression on my face.

"No sir, we don't have one, at least at this moment." I replied.

"You should have it doctor." He insisted.

"Is it that important?"

"Yes. I have a gift for you today."

"Gift? What gift?" I asked with a surprised look on my face.

He smiled and took out a small plastic bag from his pocket and kept it on the coffee table.

Everyone looked at the bag with curiosity on their faces.

"Can I see this?" I asked.

"By all means, this is in fact for you."

With my curiosity heightened, I took the closed small plastic bag and looked at it carefully. I found some small crawling insects inside it.

"I see some crawling insects inside it sir." I said.

"You are perfectly right."

"Where did you get them?" I asked.

He relaxed and leaned back in his chair, stretched his legs under the table and answered, "This is very interesting Dr. Potdar."

"What is that?"

"Now please listen all of you." He started narrating the story.

"Yesterday when we finished our work at five in the evening, I was tired. So I decided to go for a stroll on the lawn outside the plant. I saw some heaps of cut grass all along the sides of the road within the factory premises. Just out of curiosity I looked at those heaps. I saw some movement in it. My curiosity increased and I began to examine the heap more closely. To my big surprise I found these small crawling insects in the heaps of cut grass. In fact there were quite a few. Luckily I had a small plastic bag in my pocket which I keep to keep the chewing gum. Today when I came in the morning and was entering your pharma plant I saw these same insects crawling onto the steps of the building. The heaps of cut grass were still lying on the sides of the road. Do you know what this means?"

"What?"

"Those insects had sufficient time to cross the road and enter the pharma plant because the heaps of cut grass were lying on the side of the road since yesterday four in the evening to nine in the morning today."

"Oh my god!" I exclaimed, "We will take immediate corrective action about this sir."

"That is not enough Doctor, I think you should look into the following things:

1. Have some pest control for your lawns immediately so that such insects will not be there at any time.

2. The mowed grass should be immediately removed and destroyed, preferably by incineration.

3. The garden supervisor should be trained to look after not only the lawns but all other vegetation in the factory to ensure that there are no such pests in the garden.

This is a very serious issue. In my opinion it is critical observation."

"I understand sir. I will immediately call my horticulturist and give him appropriate instructions. I will also arrange for getting an SOP on lawn mowing and train the concerned people in this. I will have the SOP ready and show it you by today evening." I put forward my explanation.

He nodded his head.

It was definitely a critical issue but he recognised the sincerity of our desire to fix the problem and so thanks to his understanding nature he did not put the observation as "critical."

But remember that sometimes we think certain issues are minor but they can snowball into a crisis. You need to be very careful and should never take anything for granted.

68

INSPECTION OF LABELLING MACHINE

The same TGA audit, had a lady inspector in the team. She was auditing the injectable department on the second day of inspection. She spent nearly four hours since morning going over each and every activity related to the manufacturing of injectibles.

Incidentally no adverse observations were made by her. We were very happy, and she said, "I am very happy. Things seem to be in good shape here."

"Thanks ma'am. " I said.

We had our lunch and then she wanted to see one completed BPCR of the injectable product. This was immediately arranged for. We were sitting in my office in the main building. Only two of us were there and she was going through the BPCR very carefully.

After forty to forty five minutes she said, "Doctor Potdar, can we have a look at your injection labelling operations?"

"Why not?" I said and we moved from the main administrative building to the injectable manufacturing plant again.

"I would like to see the ampoule labelling activity, if it is ON," she said.

"Let me check if the activity is going on now or if they have finished for the day." I said and we went into the packaging hall where the injection labelling machine was installed.

I saw the operator had just finished the work and was trying to dismantle the parts.

"Ma'am the activity is just finished. Do you have anything specific in mind?" I asked her.

"Please ask the operator to stop dismantling for a while and get me the packaging record of this batch." She said.

The supervisor came to us with the document. She carefully looked into the reconciliation records of the ampoule labels and asked the supervisor to explain the same to her.

The supervisor was very smart. His mathematics was perfect and he showed how many labels he received, how many got spoiled, how many were used for the ampoules and everything. The balance sheet was perfect to 100% and he was very happy. But the lady was not. At least we could not see the satisfaction on her face.

Now she called the operator and asked him to dismantle the machine and clean it in her presence. He started to do that.

He kept the gum pot in one tray and the other parts in another tray.

"Can you wash this gum pot first and then proceed with the other things?" She asked.

I explained to the operator to wash the gum pot first. He ran to get the water. He poured the water in the pot, washed it with his hand and drained the contents in the tray.

The supervisor did not understand what she was looking for. But I got an idea of what she wanted to prove.

When the operator washed the gum pot we found about 6 to 7 labels in the tray.

"Tell me gentlemen, your reconciliation is 100% correct mathematically, but I did not see any account of these labels in your document. How is that?" She asked the supervisor.

He did not have any answer.

"Your document is forged. Am I right?"

He still did not have any answer.

"You are right ma'am." I came to his rescue.

"Please gentlemen, do not reconcile your packaging material to 100% by forgery. It really does not matter if it is 99.9 %. It is okay. Acceptable. But forging gives a wrong impression about your attitude. It is not only about this particular incident but also every other activity that you are involved in. Am I right?"

"Yes ma'am. Sorry ma'am. I will take your advice in the right spirit and avoid such things in the future," the supervisor said.

"Okay, thanks."

We left the scene.

The lesson from this incident is that never try to forge things and never take the other person for granted. The other person may be a lot wiser than you think.

69

HAIR IN TABLET

"**D**r. Potdar, can you come into my room for a minute?" Dr. Prakash Khasgiwal was on the other side. Dr. Khasgiwal was Quality and R and D Head of Plethico and I was looking after manufacturing.

"Of course, any problem Doctor?"

"Somewhat, but if you come, it will be nice."

"Sure." I was sitting just next to his room in our Indore city plant of Plethico. Incidentally Plethico had three plants one in the city, one in Mangalia and one in Kalaria.

"Yes doctor, what is the problem?" I asked Dr. Khasgiwal as I entered his room.

"Come sit down. See, this tablet batch which was under compression has some hair in it." Dr. Khasgiwal showed me some tablets lying in a petri dish on his table.

I carefully looked at those tablets, scratching my head. He was right. There was hair in it.

"Yes." I said.

"You know Manohar, this batch was started in the morning, four drums were compressed in the morning which showed no hair contamination. But the two drums which were compressed in the afternoon showed this problem. We checked the granules, but it did not show any hair in it. I don't know what is this mystery."

"Shall we go down again and check?" I asked.

"No point, I have seen everything and I have collected samples from each drum and also the granules. All these samples were collected by Nandu."

"Nandu must have done a perfect job."

"Yes."

"On the way I had a word with Babuji (our M.D.). He called us to his room. So I thought before we go there you should know the issue."

"Good, so shall we go to him?"

"Yes. I think so. " Dr. Khasgiwal got all the sample bags with him.

" Give them to me sir. I will take them." I said.

"It is alright Manohar." Dr. Khasgiwal said as we were leaving the room.

"Good morning Babuji." We said.

"Good morning. Come, come. Could you get any clue about the hair?" Babuji asked us.

"Not really" we both said.

"Hmm sit down." We occupied the chairs in front of him.

" Prakash show me those tablets in the sequence in which they were compressed." Dr. Khasgiwal showed the plastic bags which were numbered 1, 2, 3, 4, 5 and 6 and a bag of granules.

"So the first four bags show no hair and they were compressed before lunch. Is it?"

"Yes sir." Dr. Khasgiwal said.

"And the bags five and six were compressed after lunch?"

"Yes sir."

"Manohar can you call the operator?"

"Yes sir." I sent a message to the ground floor to call the tablet machine operator.

"May I come in sir?," the operator Santosh Kumar sought permission to enter.

"Yes come in Santosh."

"Namaste sir." Santosh greeted Babuji with a little worry on his face. Santosh Kumar was an experienced reliable and skilled operator.

"Santosh are you aware of the problem with the tablets today?" Babuji asked him.

"Yes sir. It has never happened in the past sir. I really don't know what went wrong. Believe me sir."

"Okay tell me what you did after lunch."

"Sir I did not have lunch today as I am fasting."

"Okay. Then what did you do in the lunch time?"

"Sir for the last four days I have been working overtime in the evening right up to nine o' clock."

"So?"

"I was planning to get a haircut for the past week but I wasn't able to find any time."

"Then?"

"Sir today I was fasting so I thought I could get my hair cut during the lunch time since the barber's shop is close by."

"Then what did you do?"

"I had the hair cut sir and came back in time sir. It took just twenty minutes."

"Good, Santosh you can remove your cap, it is not necessary to wear it in my office."

Santosh removed his cap and held it in his hand.

"Come here for a moment Santosh." Babuji asked Santosh.

Santosh looked at us in a puzzled manner.

"Show me your cap."

Santosh showed the cap to Babuji.

Babuji looked inside the cap and passed it to Dr. Khasgiwal and Dr. Khasgiwal looked at it and then passed it to me.

The inside of the cap had a lot of cut hair in it.

"Prakash, this is the culprit. The hair cut."

"Your guess is right sir."

"Not my guess. It is reason, you know?"

"Yes sir."

"Santosh your hair cut has spoilt our two drums of tablets. Aapko samaj main aayi aapki galti kya hai?"

"Yes sir, I am very sorry sir. I should not have gone for my hair cut while on duty."

"You are right. Now go straight to your home and do not even enter the production area. Understand?"

"Yes sir."

"And never make such a mistake again."

"Never sir."

"Go." Babuji said.

"This is the mystery Manohar. You need to train your boys on all such matters then only you will be able to avoid such gross mistakes."

"I understand sir." I said.

"Good."

"Thank you sir."

"Prakash reject those last two drums and Manohar get the previous drums also checked hundred percent before Prakash takes any appropriate decision on it. Is that clear?"

"Yes sir." We said and left his room.

"Manohar, have we ever learnt this in our BITS Pilani?" Dr. Khasgiwal asked me.

"You never taught this to us sir." I said, with a naughty smile.

Incidentally Dr. Prakash Chandra Khasgiwal was my teacher in BITS Pilani. Both of us were Pilani products. That was when we realised that college education has its limitations.

70

MCC Audit at Plethico

It was at about 4:00 P.M. in the evening, my telephone on the table rang.

"Hello"

"Dr. Potdar, I have called for a meeting in my office at 6:00 P.M. today. Please come without fail."

"Yes sir." I replied.

I knew that our director Babuji was scheduled to leave the next day to U.S for his medical check-up. His brother was a cardiologist and a surgeon in the U.S. I thought Babuji was calling me because he was not going to be in Indore for some time. I was in the Kalaria plant at that time.

I was just thinking about the meeting and the phone rang again.

"Hello." I responded.

"Doctor I am Khasgiwal speaking."

"Sir."

"Babuji has called a meeting at 6:00 P.M. in his office. Did you get a call from him?"

"Yes sir, I am reaching there before 6:00 P.M."

"That is good. Mr. Rao (our Manglia plant Head) and I will reach at about five thirty. If you could join us in my office before the meeting; that would be nice."

"No problem sir." I replied to Dr. Khasgiwal.

At five thirty we met in Dr. Khasgiwal's room and identified if any points need to be discussed with Babuji in the meeting and then left together for the meeting in Babuji's room.

Babuji welcomed us all and ordered for some tea and biscuits.

"Good that you are all here." He said as he took out a letter from his drawer and said, "Prakash, today we have received this letter from M.C.C. South Africa. They have scheduled our audit after ten days. This is for you Manglia plant Mr. Rao." Babuji gave the letter to Dr. Prakash Khasgiwal.

"Fine sir." Mr. Rao said.

"I know for certain time is very short. Even though we know the audit can be at any time, yet ten days is a very short notice for an M.C.C audit, but we have no choice."

"Yes sir, the time is short, but don't worry. We will do our best." I said.

"Dr. Potdar I know that you will do your best. I have full confidence in you people, but the task is very difficult and challenging." Babuji expressed his opinion.

"Yes sir." All of us said simultaneously.

"I have thought on this and I have some suggestions. They are just suggestions and the final decision will be yours."

"Yes sir, what do you have in mind?" Dr. Khasgiwal asked.

"Prakash, I repeat this is only my suggestion."

"Yes sir." Dr. Khasgiwal responded.

"Prakash you will form a team of four people and you will be heading the team and Dr. Potdar, Mr. Rao and Suresh Pardeshi (who was our chief engineer) will be the other team members."

"Okay sir."

"Prakash you will take care of all Quality Management related issues. Rao will see that Manglia plant operations are up to date and Dr. Potdar can take care of all documentation, validation etc. and also can take care of the two auditors who are coming from M.C.C South Africa. Your responsibilities start from the moment they land at the Indore airport till you see them off from there after three or four days, as the case may be. Is that clear?" Babuji asked.

"No problem sir." I said.

"Second thing, I have already instructed Mr. Mody (our finance head) about keeping sufficient cash handy, since the time is short you may need some cash for some sundry purchases and all. In my absence Prakash you will have the authority to get any finances required from Mr. Mody. I have told him to honour any request from you."

"Yes sir." Dr. Khasgiwal said.

"Now the last thing, I am leaving for Mumbai tomorrow. I have a flight from there at midnight. I know the job is not simple, but if we get the approval the entire credit will go to you and your team. If we fail I will not be surprised because I know for certain that the time is short for such an international audit. We will always have a second chance. Okay?"

"Yes sir."

"If we get through, Prakash give me a call to the U.S, if not don't worry. We will see what we can do afterwards when I come back to Indore after about a month or so. Best of luck boys." Babuji said while picking up his jacket from the hanger. We got up, the meeting was over. The peon opened the door of Babuji's cabin with Babuji's briefcase in hand. Babuji got down the stairs and we followed him.

"Manohar we have to meet tomorrow right in the morning at 8. Rao you don't go to the plant directly, come here to my office and then maybe we can go to the plant together after the meeting is over.

Manohar please call Suresh too here for the meeting tomorrow morning." Dr. Khasgiwal said.

"Yes sir." I assured him.

We attended the meeting the next day in Dr. Khasgiwals office. A detailed strategy was worked out. Some of the key points other than what Babuji had told us the previous day were:

1. Indore city plant and the Kalaria plant will be looked after by the number two people in the plant and Dr. Khasgiwal, Suresh Pardeshi and I will be fully concentrating on Manglia plant where the M.C.C inspection was scheduled.

2. Any additional manpower required for Manglia plant will be provided by the other two plants. This will include supervisory, managerial as well as workers.

3. No person from Manglia plant will be granted leave, unless and until an extreme emergency demands and that will be with prior sanction of Mr. Rao, who was the works manager of the plant.

4. No one would leave the Manglia plant without Mr. Rao's permission.

After the meeting was over we all reached the Manglia plant at about ten thirty in the morning. Immediately at eleven a meeting of the supervisory and managerial staff was called and Mr. Rao gave a complete picture of the audit and related issues to the group. He also explained the immediate needs and the points which were discussed in the morning meeting.

After this the department heads were told to communicate this news to all the workmen and motivate them and accept this as a challenge for the Manglia plant.

With all this preparatory work we ourselves got motivated and were self-confident about the audit.

Dr. Khasgiwal suggested that we should not spend any more time in meetings and instead we should get started with our individual responsibilities amongst the four of us i.e., Rao, Suresh, myself and Dr. Khasgiwal himself.

It was also agreed that once in a day preferably at about four in the evening we four would meet to discuss the progress and issues if any.

You will not believe for the next ten days everyone in the plant right from the sweeper to Dr. Khasgiwal worked furiously, with only one aim, that we must succeed in this M.C.C audit. Remember that these plant people did not have any previous exposure to any international audit such as this one. The only audit they had faced was by W.H.O.

While having a cup of tea in Mr. Rao's cabin, I was planning my own strategy about my work. I tried a new concept of **"Small area complete responsibility"**. This was my own idea. I was not sure about whether it would work or not but I planned and executed it.

Small Area Complete Responsibility Concept

This concept was something like this – I had about fifteen supervisors and executives in the manufacturing department i.e., production and warehousing.

What I did was physically, you may call it geographically also if you want, divided the entire auditable plant into fifteen areas e.g.,

- Granulation I
- Granulation II
- Compression section
- Strip packaging
- Blister packaging
- Garden and lawns etc.

Each of the supervisors was given charge of each of these single areas. Engineering people kept away from this, since they had to do many other activities and also support the people in manufacturing units.

Each of the fifteen supervisors I took with me individually, accompanied him to his area and audited that small area in complete detail and identified:

- Deficiencies in that area are noted and also decided on how these deficiencies can be overcomed.

- Made a list of certain questions that the auditors may ask in this area.

- Provided them the M.C.C South Africa guide lines and asked them to study in the next four or five days, so that they are equipped with a basic understanding of the audit.

The area responsibility included every aspect of the audit in the given area like:

- Facilities – painting, maintenance, light, etc.

- Equipment – cleaning, validation reports, maintenance reports, history cards, etc.

- People – Training records, leave records, uniform, medical check-up reports, etc.

- Document – MPCR/ BPCR, SOP, exhibited SOPs, various production reports.

- IPQC etc.

In short each of these areas in-charge, could be a supervisor, officer or at the most executive. The selection was preferably from their own areas and he was to work like a 'works manager' of that small domain and he had the complete responsibility of that area to make it totally 'deficiency free'.

This concept of "complete responsibility" highly motivated these youngsters. Not only this, but they also came to know about what is the overall scope of the audit activity. Also the fifteen youngsters got an opportunity to demonstrate their leadership qualities and each of these units became a self-contained unit in all respects from the audit point of view.

The biggest advantage of this concept was that senior managers got enough free time to attend to many other important activities which only they can do.

Two days after I initiated and kicked off the system, I explained this concept in our core meeting (i.e. the small group of Mr. Rao, Mr. Suresh and Dr. Khasgiwal.) They liked the idea and Dr. Khasgiwal initiated the same in his Q.C. lab as well.

The second new idea was initiated by our chief engineer, Mr. Suresh Pardeshi. This was implemented during the audit itself.

I will briefly explain what he did.

On day of the audit which started at about eleven in the morning, after the initial welcome, company presentation etc. Mr. Pardeshi requested me to hire a photographer for two days which I did.

The auditors were accompanied by Mr. Rao, Dr. Khasgiwal, the photographer and me. Whenever the auditors pointed out a physical deficiency he used to click a picture of that and pass on the information to Mr. Suresh Pardeshi. Suresh had a team of maintenance people ready with him, he would ensure that the physical deficiency would be immediately taken care of, as the auditors moved to the next area.

This activity went on the whole day and Suresh tried to take care of say 80 % of the deficiencies that day and also during the night by keeping his people on their toes.

After the deficiency was corrected he would snap another picture of the corrected situation in the night itself and he will make an album of the deficiencies as pointed out by the auditors and the corrective action taken on them by the plant management. Under each photograph he wrote the description of the deficiency along with the room name, number and time and at the side of this he will paste the corrected situation photograph.

If there was some deficiency which could not be corrected in a day he would make a note beside the photograph of when this particular deficiency would be corrected.

He carried the album with him, when on day 2 we met for tea in the morning before the start of the audit on the second day.

When Mr. Westhousen the senior M.C.C inspector was having tea Mr. Pardeshi showed him the album, which was very well prepared, and said,

"Sir this album shows what deficiencies you have pointed out yesterday and what actions we have taken to correct them over night."

Mr. Westhousen had a look at that and got literally excited about this approach.

"My god, Mr. Pardeshi hats off to you. I never expected this type of action, which is unusual, quick, and very systematic. If you permit me I would like to carry this album with me to my office." Westhousen explained.

"Why not sir, in fact this is for you." Pardeshi said. We all looked towards Pardeshi with a surprised look on our face but an appreciating smile on our faces.

The second day went very smoothly. At about four in the evening, the older inspector told me, "Doctor, I will have a look at your new purified water plant tomorrow, right in the morning."

"No problem sir." I assured him.

While I assured him that he can have a look at the new water system in the morning, I realised that a very serious problem was in. The drain connection from the water system to the ETP was not yet made and we had told the auditors that the system is fully operational. This statement was totally incorrect and I was worried.

I called Suresh and explained the situation to him and asked him to go and see what could be done to save the situation tomorrow.

Suresh came after half an hour.

"Sir don't worry, I will do it for you. You can bring the inspector at 9:00 A.M. tomorrow. No problem." Suresh told me.

"What will you do Suresh? The drain pipe is not made and it is not possible to build it overnight." I said.

"What to do is my problem. You please don't ask me how. But I assure you only one thing, tomorrow you will not have any problem." Suresh assured me with confidence.

"Okay. I will not ask. But he will be here right in the morning. Please remember that and do whatever you can." I closed the matter.

"Okay sir, can I go now? I have some other problems that I need to attend to."

"Okay." I said. Suresh left to attend to his pressing problems.

"After tea we will go straight to the purified water treatment plant." The inspector reminded me.

"Okay sir." I said.

I called Suresh and told him that we will be there after tea. Suresh confirmed me that he has done everything required and I should not worry about it.

The water treatment plant was a little away from the main plant and the ETP was behind the water treatment plant.

We had our tea and left the main plant office and started walking towards the water treatment plant.

"Good morning sir." Suresh greeted the inspector on the way as we walked. Suresh had a mischievous smile on his face but I could not guess the exact reason behind it.

"Good morning." The inspector reciprocated.

We entered the water treatment plant, the inspector checked everything very carefully and finally asked the question which I never wanted him to ask.

"Suresh what happens to the acid base washed drain?"

"Sir please come behind the plant, I will show you the drain system." We all walked behind.

There was a pipe coming out from the plant and going into the soil below.

"The drained washings come in this pipe from the plant which you have just seen and there is an underground pipe and going from here to that ETP which you see." Suresh showed the boundary wall of the ETP receiving tank.

"Oh good, good, good," said the inspector.

I thought the inspection is over.

"Can I have a look at that receiving tank?"

Now I got really scared, because I knew that we had not done any connection to this.

"Why not sir? Please come." Suresh said.

I was totally surprised.

Suresh took us both to the ETP tank. The inspector literally stepped upon the wall of the tank carefully holding onto the grills around that wall.

Suresh accompanied him and both of them looked below onto the other side. They talked something and then Suresh got down and helped the inspector to get down. I was waiting a little away from the wall.

"Good that is fine." The M.C.C inspector remarked when he came back. He was satisfied.

The third day of the inspection went smoothly. After lunch on the third day Mr. Westhousen said they are happy and the inspection is through.

The auditors left the next day. I saw them off and then returned to the factory.

I reached my office and picked up my intercom. "Hello Suresh."

"Yes sir."

"Please come into my room immediately."

"Yes sir I am coming. In fact I was waiting for you, I am just coming." Suresh said.

"Hello sir." Suresh entered my room.

"Come, come Suresh."

"How is everything sir? The guests have gone back safely?"

"Yes very safely."

"That's good. We must have a party from you sir, the inspection went smoothly." Suresh was excited.

"You will, but I am puzzled about one small thing Suresh."

"What's that sir?"

"Tell me how did you manage the drainage system from the WTP to the ETP over night? We did not even have any material at hand." I asked.

"I was expecting this question from you sir."

"Tell me what magic wand you have with you?"

"Trade secret sir, I hope you will not tell this to anyone and certainly not fire me."

"Don't tell me all that. Tell me what exactly did you do and how?"

"Sir I did nothing, in fact I had only two pipes with me of say about two meters and some 'L' joints of the same size."

"So what did you do with that?"

"I took only one boy with me Moti Singh with me, you know him very well."

"I know, what did you do then?"

"Sir, I fixed one pipe from the outlet of the WTP with an 'L' joint and buried that pipe in the ground outside the WTP and the other pipe dipped in the receiver tank of ETP which already had some water so the pipe got dipped inside the receiving tank."

"And how did you join that long link underground?"

"Now I am going to get a beating from you, I know."

"What do you mean?"

"Sir actually I did not lay any connecting pipe between WTP and ETP. There was nothing there underground. Even today also there is nothing there. But I have planned to do that work in the next two days one hundred percent Sir." Suresh told me.

"What are you telling me Suresh? Tell me what you would have done if he had asked to see the connection?' I asked completely aghast.

"It was the biggest risk I took sir."

"Thank god we were lucky. But just tell me what would you have done had we been exposed."

"Surrendered, I would have accepted that it is my fault and no one else is responsible for that."

"Suresh please, for god's sake never take such a risk in your life ever again."

"I know sir I will not. But when you told me the situation yesterday this was the only possible solution I could come up with. I am really sorry sir."

"Hmmm okay."

The peon brought in two cups of tea. We had the first sip of the days with a completely relaxed body and mind.

Babuji must be waiting for our call. I picked up my intercom and asked the operator to connect me to Babuji in the U.S.

71

THE BLACK DIWALI

Sometimes we face some tragic situations in the industry. These situations can be avoided if we take a little care in the safety practices of the factory.

One such even took place in the factory where I was working.

We used to use some inflammable solvents during the process of manufacturing. We used to receive these solvent in 200 litres steel drums. These drums use to be very good for storage of water in the houses of employees.

Whenever the drums were empty they were transferred to our scrap yards and these were sold to the employees at nominal cost.

On the previous day of our Diwali holiday one of the security guards purchased a drum for himself and took it home. The next day was the first day of Diwali.

As we understand from his family members, he brought the drum and kept outside his house that evening. The next day morning i.e. on Diwali day he wanted to fill it with water. But before filling it with water he wanted to see that the drum is completely clean. Since the water that he wanted to store in the drum was not for drinking and only for sundry purposes he did not think it was essential to wash it thoroughly before use.

The time was early morning maybe around 5 AM and he was looking into the drum. He could not see properly because it was still dark outside, so he asked his daughter to get a candle. The daughter and the guard himself did not realise the seriousness of the use of a lighted candle. She gave the candle to her father and went back inside the house. The guard probably wanted to see the cleanliness of the drum and make sure that it was free from the 'solvent' using the light of the candle. And even before he could realise what is happening the traces of solvent from the drum which would have been in vapour form exploded with a great noise and fire.

The daughter rushed outside to see what happened, she could see nothing but a totally broken drum in the fire and the most unfortunate scene was the smashed dead body of her father.

A very very unfortunate incident indeed.

When we came to know about this the following actions were taken:

1. The daughter of the guard was provided a job in the company. She was just an eighteen year old, twelfth standard passed girl. This gave the family some financial support.

2. An SOP was developed and immediately implemented to safely handle the empty solvent drums. One of the main points in this SOP was to wash the empty solvent drums with plenty of water and keep them open for drying and when dried, to be sent to the scrap yard.

72

THE PROJECT MEETING

It was the 20th or 21st of October 2003 and I was in the Alkem's Head Office in Mumbai to attend a meeting on a new project with the M.D and Chairman along with other functional heads.

The meeting lasted only ten minutes in which the chairman said, "We are starting a new project in Baddi, Himachal Pradesh, where we have a piece of land purchased and ready. I want the factory to be ready and dispatch the first truck of finished goods in April 2005. So far you are confident to meet this requirement within the specified budget and meeting the current quality requirements for a pharmaceutical plant, I do not want to receive any frequent reports. Any questions?"

The unanimous answer was "NO QUESTIONS SIR."

I was sure the old man (Affectionate name for the chairman) knew the importance of project Management and believe me he supported the entire project team and we were able to dispatch the first truck of finished goods on 14th April, 2005 in his presence. I was only the project leader but the credit goes to the entire team.

The project management had a three way target, it has to focus on time, cost and quality performance.

73

MONITORING MEN IN STERILE FILLING

It was in Jan 2005, when our Alkem plant at Daman was undergoing MHRA approval audit.

Mr. John Clark was one of the auditors. The audit was only for sterile products facility.

Practically everything went off smoothly in the audit. But in any audit there is always at least one thing that goes wrong and the same thing happened here.

Mr. John Clark, Mr. Ravi Pandey (He was the Vice-President of Production) and I were walking through the corridor from where we could easily see the sterile filling operations. John stopped near the double glass window through which we could see the sterile filling operations. The filling machine was practically in the centre of the room and provided with an LAF unit and was closed from the sides with flexible plastic. The operator was in a "cover-all" sterile garment. John observed the operation with full concentration for more than ten minutes standing in the corridor looking through the double glass window.

The operator kept intervening the process by intermediately putting his hand through the plastic curtain.

"Tell me Potdar, you monitor the operator on which class of air?" John asked me.

"As class 10,000 sir" I responded.

"Class 10,000?"

"Yes sir."

"The filling is under class hundred, is it not?"

"You are right sir."

"And the operator is monitored at class 10,000?"

"You are right again sir."

"Don't you see anything wrong in this?"

"Why sir?"

"Tell me why do you monitor him as per class 10,000?"

"John, he is standing I mean operating from a class 10,000 area."

"But he puts his hand in to the class 100 area at times."

"I know that, but all the time he is in a class 10,000 area and only sometimes he puts a small part of his body, that is his forehand into the class 100 area. That's why we monitor him as a class 10,000 area person." I explained.

"No I don't accept this justification. Because if he is intervening in class 100, maybe rarely and maybe a very small part of his body, but according to me he is interfering with class 100 area and therefore must be monitored as per class 100 area."

Ravi and I looked at each other with a question mark on our faces.

"It is a critical observation Dr Potdar." John continued.

I looked at him a little dissatisfied.

"Don't you agree with me Dr. Potdar?"

"I agree but so far we have been monitoring him as a class 10,000"

"You need to do something in this regard." John insisted.

"Yes John, we will do it. Ravi please call Onkar on the way to my office after 5 minutes."

"Sir." Ravi called Onkar our Q.A Head and we went back to my room from there. Onkar reached my office within no time at all.

I explained the whole situation to Onkar and asked him to make an SOP revision of the person monitoring from class 10,000 to class 100.

We showed the SOP to Mr. John Clark and said that we would train the monitoring people as per this SOP and implement it with immediate effect. However nothing can be done about what we have been doing till now.

"John I think since we have accepted your suggestion and are going to implement it with immediate effect, you should take a lenient view on this observation and not write it as critical." I requested John.

"Hmmm I think since there is no other adverse observation I will not put this in critical category, but I would like to see the revised SOP by today evening."

"No problem John. We will certainly do it."

He agreed. Sometimes we have our own thinking, but the auditors think otherwise. My opinion is that if you show a concern for their views they will generally accept your views if they see that you are genuine.

74

THE MISTY ISSUE

It was the occasion of MHRA audit at Alkem Daman plant. The dates were Jan 4, 5 and 6th of 2004.

The first day of inspection went very smoothly. I was very happy. The next day they were to proceed with sterile products manufacturing and utility support services for this department i.e. HVAC, water, gases, etc. The audit was to start early at 8:00 o' clock in the morning and I was supposed to bring the auditors from the hotel Miramar.

I got ready early and was to leave my house and go to the hotel Miramar to pick up the auditors and take them to the factory. It was about 7:30 A.M or so and I came out of my house and saw to my surprise that there was heavy mist; the entire area was dense and foggy. So much so that it was impossible to even see twenty feet ahead. The visibility was extremely poor and my driver with the car was waiting outside.

"Sir today there is very dense fog and the visibility is very very poor. I came all the way with the headlights on and yet I had to drive very very slowly." My driver told me.

"Yes, I can see that. We have to go to hotel Miramar on beach road. We have to go slowly and keep the head lights on." I said.

"Don't worry sir I will drive safely."

"Okay, just wait I will come within five minutes."

I went inside put on my shoes, took the briefcase and came outside.

"Shall we go sir?"

"Yes." I said sitting in the car.

The driver was driving the car very slowly and cautiously. It was already 8 o'clock when we reached Miramar. I got out of the car and was entering the hotel reception when my mobile rang.

"Hello."

"Hello sir, I am Ravi speaking." It was my VP of production on the line.

"Yes Ravi?"

"Sir we have a little problem."

"What's that?"

"Sir please speak to the chief engineer Anil."

"Yes Anil is there any problem?"

"Sir there is a major electric failure. The main supply has tripped. My boys are already on the job and are working on the sub-station transformer. We will be able to fix it by 9 o'clock or so. Maybe even before that. But still till such time we fix it the plant is entirely shut down and I do not want to start the DG set now for some reasons which I will explain to you later." Anil said in a worried voice.

"So what do you want from me right now?"

"Sir please delay the visit of the auditors till 9 o'clcok. I will surely fix the problem till then."

"Okay" I said.

I entered the reception and checked whether the guests were in their rooms or in the restaurant having breakfast. The receptionist checked and told me that they were in the restaurant having breakfast.

I went to the restaurant which was on the ground floor facing the sea.

"Good morning John."

"Good morning Dr. Potdar. What is the climate today? Suddenly it is so misty."

"Yes we were also finding it very difficult to drive." I said.

"Would you like to have something?" John asked me.

"I will have a cup of coffee." I said and asked for a cup of coffee from the waiter. I did not know how to delay these people from going to the factory. Suddenly I got an idea.

"John, you have breakfast and stay in your room, meanwhile I will check the latest police warnings about the fog."

"What is that warning."

"In the morning the chief of police gave a warning to avoid vehicular traffic to avoid accidents."

"Oh my god! Is it?"

"Yes, I too did not know about this. On the way the constable told us to stay off the road and I told him that I will be parking my car in the near-by hotel and managed to come here." I plainly bluffed.

"Oh that is really good police service in the town." John praised our Daman police.

John and the other inspectors had their breakfast and went back to their rooms and I was waiting in the reception.

The fog slowly started cleaned by about 8:45 and the visibility was fairly good. I checked with Anil the status of the electrical failure and he gave me the green signal.

I went to John's room.

"John, I think we can move, the fog has cleaned now." I said.

"What about the police warning?"

"Now since the visibility is good, I don't think there will be a problem."

"Good then we can move." John said.

We came down and left for the factory and in the factory everything was fixed up properly and we were ready for any type of inspection now.

"Thank you sir." Anil whispered in my ears.

"Thanks to the mist Anil, it helped us." I said while entering the conference room with the auditors.

"Sometimes nature helps us. You will ask me what would have happened if the inspectors had come when there is no electricity in the factory".

A good question.

We can always explain the thing to them but this may lead to many unwanted issues like validation of electrical failure, how do you validate the filling and sterilisation process during such electrical failure and many more.

We can of course always have appropriate answers for such questions, but my personal suggestion is that if you can avoid such tricky situations then please avoid them.

75

DEDICATION TO
WORK - MANAGING BY STYLE

You will always get examples of various human qualities in personal life and also in your industrial life. Dedication is one of the important human qualities and in the industry too you find some people exhibiting this quality.

Here I am giving an example of what exactly dedication is.

It was the second day of our MHRA inspection. The last day was already really hectic but thankfully the things were going smoothly. It was about 7:00 P.M. in the evening and the auditors had already gone to the hotel and we were planning for the next and final day of work when my intercom rang,

"Sir are you free for a few minute, I have to discuss something with you urgently." Mr. Onkar Nath Singh was on the other line.

"Yes Onkar, come down please."

Onkar entered my room.

"Yes Onkar?"

"Sir I have a small issue related to our microbiology testing."

"Okay. Let us see what that is." I talked to Onkar and we discussed the matter for about twenty minutes.

I observed that Onkar was not alright and his eyes were heavy, he looked quite tired and exhausted.

"Onkar are you alright?" I asked him touching his hand. His hand was literally hot. I got up from my chair and touched his forehead. He was running a high temperature.

"Onkar, you are running a high fever." I said.

"Yes sir, I have taken a paracetamol tablet sometime back. I think it will subside."

"Are you mad? You go home immediately. Take my driver and don't bother about tomorrow I will manage with your boys. Take rest tomorrow I think most of the audit is almost completed. Even if it is not, you don't come. Ravi and I will take care."

"Anyway I am leaving now sir, I think it will be okay by tomorrow." Onkar said.

"Onkar you are not coming tomorrow. You need complete rest. Okay?"

I called my driver and asked him to drive Onkar home.

On the third and final day of the inspection I asked Ravi to come in early and look into the Q.C lab as Onkar would not be there.

I entered the factory with John and the other inspector and we went straight to my room. I made arrangements for a cup of tea for the auditors and rushed to the Q.C Lab to see that the things were in shape.

When I entered the lab, I saw to my big surprise Onkar sitting at his table on his chair with some of his colleagues to whom he was giving instructions. I was shocked.

"Onkar? You are here?" I asked.

"Yes sir." He had a pleasant smile on his face and continued, "Sir, I thought I would take the day off tomorrow, instead of today. Today I will manage. I know you and Ravi would have definitely managed today's Q.C Audit but then I thought it would be too taxing for you and Ravi both, since you have many other things to look after. I am okay sir. There is slight weakness but manageable. Sir you can be with the auditors and please don't worry about anything here. Everything is in it's place. We will meet after the audit today. I am sure we will get through and you will owe us all a party." Onkar was confident.

I put my hand affectionately on his head and said,

"Okay take care. I am in my office with John." And I left the room.

This is what is called dedication to work. With such an attitude I am sure Onkar will achieve the highest success in life.